The Psychology and Communication Behind Flight Anxiety

The Psychology and Communication Behind Flight Anxiety

Afraid to Fly

Lindsey A. Harvell-Bowman

Foreword by Eric M. Wilson

LEXINGTON BOOKS
Lanham • Boulder • New York • London

Published by Lexington Books
An imprint of The Rowman & Littlefield Publishing Group, Inc.
4501 Forbes Boulevard, Suite 200, Lanham, Maryland 20706
www.rowman.com

6 Tinworth Street, London SE11 5AL, United Kingdom

British Library Cataloguing in Publication Information Available

Library of Congress Cataloging-in-Publication Data Available

ISBN 978-1-7936-2069-9 (cloth)
ISBN 978-1-7936-2070-5 (electronic)

The Psychology and Communication Behind Flight Anxiety

Afraid to Fly

Lindsey A. Harvell-Bowman

Foreword by Eric M. Wilson

LEXINGTON BOOKS
Lanham • Boulder • New York • London

Published by Lexington Books
An imprint of The Rowman & Littlefield Publishing Group, Inc.
4501 Forbes Boulevard, Suite 200, Lanham, Maryland 20706
www.rowman.com

6 Tinworth Street, London SE11 5AL, United Kingdom

British Library Cataloguing in Publication Information Available

Library of Congress Cataloging-in-Publication Data Available

ISBN 978-1-7936-2069-9 (cloth)
ISBN 978-1-7936-2070-5 (electronic)

*This book is dedicated to my husband,
who remarkably still chooses to sit next to me (and
even claim me as family) while on a plane.*

Contents

List of Figures and Tables

FIGURES

TABLES

List of Figures and Tables

FIGURES

TABLES

Foreword

Flying. A thoughtless routine for some. Or a means to an end. A major event or experience for others. It's a ritual that many have come to rely on and often take for granted.

Whether you view commercial flight as a technological marvel, a necessary annoyance of travel or work, or with sheer joy and wonder, flying is a shared experience. A modern convenience—and also sometimes a hassle—air travel is a lightning rod for media coverage, government regulators, and pundits, and even frequent fodder for stand-up comics and late-night talk show hosts.

Stepping onto an airplane and quickly transiting regions, time zones, or continents is something most can relate to (and also complain about), but people experience flight in different ways. For most, the biggest worry is "Will I make it to the gate in time?," "Will my flight arrive on time?," "Will I be able to get the seat I want?" or "Can I get an upgrade?" But for others, the thought of stepping onto a plane is a vastly different—and potentially terrifying—experience.

According to an October 2019 *Washington Post* report, about 40 percent of the general population reports a fear of flying on some level, and about 2.5 percent have a phobia that causes them to avoid taking to the skies if at all possible. The fear of danger, real and rational or not, leads to anxiety.

There are countless studies—several of which are discussed later in this book—that illuminate the safety of flying compared to other forms of transportation. But fear is often irrational, as apparent in this excerpt from a book about another common, often irrational, fear. As National Geographic contributor Glenn Hodges writes in *Shark* (2017, p. 84), "Though I kept swimming after (seeing the movie) *Jaws*, it was always with a vague fear that teeth could tug on my leg at any moment. Never mind that there have been only two shark bites on the Connecticut coast since 1900. Facts are never as salient as feelings."

While memories of travel experiences and traveling companions often last, the feelings associated with the flights themselves often fade into the background. But when you stop and reflect, the hurried, cramped nature of air travel itself can trigger many emotional responses—frustration, anxiousness, hurry, impatience, worry, tiredness, anticipation, and relaxation, to name a few. In a world of seemingly constantly increasing anxieties and in the midst of a global pandemic, all of these feelings are understandable.

What we may perceive as somewhat simple, routine acts require a complex series of actions—navigating crowded airport-mazes. Filing onto cramped aircraft amid throngs of other passengers. Locating your seat and hoping there is enough space to cram your belongings into an overhead bin or seat-back. Fastening your seat belt and then attempting to "sit back, relax, and enjoy your flight"—as we are so often directed by the flight crew—before hurtling through the sky in a pressurized metal tube at 500 miles per hour. All of it requires relinquishing coveted personal control, which is often at the root of anxieties and fears.

You have likely sat next to a nervous traveler or excitedly anxious first-time flier. You may offer a reassuring smile or kind word, or avoid eye contact, quickly connect your headphones, and try to hide your annoyance or frustration. If the increasingly complex process of navigating the airport and getting onto the plane does not cause anxiety in and of itself, what if there's turbulence? Invisible forces such as wind, thermals or so-called rough air, or visually spectacular clouds and storms all make flying more interesting, especially to those with motion sickness or other flight anxieties.

As a seasoned air traveler, former airline intern, and aviation enthusiast, I never worry much about turbulence—until the pilots come on the PA system and ask the flight attendants to be seated due to expected turbulence. More often than not, the bumps are minor if even felt at all. But memories of the few truly turbulent segments of flights I have experienced that have caused spilled drinks, gasps from passengers as the plane unexpectedly drops or rolls, and warnings from flight attendants to remain seated tend to be unsettling and trigger anxieties and fears—rational or otherwise. The unsettling, undulating motion triggers feelings of dread in the pit of my stomach. Even though everything turns out fine a vast majority of the time, in those brief, turbulent moments, minds are often drawn to news coverage or novels that dissect what went wrong in aviation disasters.

Flying requires an exchange of trust and control of one's surroundings, personal space, direction, and (at least perception of) safety. Terror Management Theory (TMT), which is applied in this text, helps guide understanding of the physiological and psychological effects of air travel. In this book, my friend and fellow avgeek, Dr. Lindsey A. Harvell-Bowman, examines the anxieties brought on by air travel through research combining psychology and communication theory in attempts to better understand and manage the common nerves associated with flying. A trailblazing scholar in TMT and a seasoned air traveler, Dr. Harvell-Bowman will use science and stories to explore these fears. More specifically, she employs TMT to explain why people are scared to fly, how the fears can be perpetuated, and what anxious air travelers can do to calm their nerves and have a more pleasant air travel experience.

My hope is that this work, through both narrative and academic exposition, will help you better understand the anxieties associated, and learn how it affects people's brains and what you can do to have a more positive experience on your next flight. Wishing you calm winds, blue skies, and on-time flights. See you at the airport!

Eric M. Wilson, MA
Senior Educator, Wichita State University
Elliott School of Communication
Wichita, KS, March 2021

Acknowledgments

For years I have pondered writing this book. I have bounced ideas off of so many people, that it still amazes me any time a family member or friend will knowingly board an aircraft with me in fear that I will start explaining the dangers of takeoff and landing. Trust me, a lot of people are happy this book is now out in the world. No one is happier than my golden retriever, who listened to countless out-loud readings of this manuscript, and always listened with great interest. I finished this book holed up in a secluded house on the shores of the James River in Virginia in the summer of 2020. I'm so incredibly grateful for those long walks on the beach with my dog wondering if I really did need that semicolon or not. And, a special thanks to my mom, who served as one of my editors, and who also surprisingly continues to fly all over the world with me, prefacing most flights with, "If we are going to crash, I don't want to know. Seriously, not a word." I hope you all enjoy reading this as much as I enjoyed writing it. Happy flying!

Credits

Quote and Figure/Table permissions provided by the following:

Dr. Martin N. Seif, Dr. Sheldon Solomon, Richard Quest, Will Self, Dr. Jamie Arndt, Dr. Alexander Lancaster, and Dr. Palmira Faraci.

Louise Thaden, excerpt from *High, Wide and Frightened.* Copyright 1938 by Louise Thaden. Copyright © 2004 by The University of Arkansas Press. Reprinted with the permission of The Permissions Company, LLC on behalf of the publishers, www.uapress.com.

Chapter 1

Flight Anxiety

Why Should We Be Worried?

Fear of flying is a feeling. Feelings aren't facts.

—Dr. Martin Seif, Clinical Psychologist

"Anxiety is the reaction to danger" (Freud, 1936, p. 93). This statement written decades ago by psychologist Sigmund Freud still stands true today. The statement seems simple enough—do not put yourself in a dangerous situation, and your anxiety should be alleviated. However, what happens when danger is not imminent, and it is simply the *fear* of danger that leads to anxiety? Fear that is not immediate can often lead to the type of anxiety that is present when individuals exhibit a fear of flying, with the worst cases being psychologically diagnosed as aviophobia.

Since flying has become more mainstream in the 1960s to 1980s, crowded airports, airplanes, and skies allow for more anxiety among passengers. Nearly one in three adults (women are twice as likely as men to have this anxiety) are either anxious about flying (18.1%) or afraid to fly (12.6%) (Davis, 2019). With the increase in air disasters over the years (e.g., MH370, Germanwings 9525, MH17, etc.), there is no reason to believe the fear of flying is improving. These fears can manifest from thinking about anything from mechanical problems (73%), bad weather (62%), or even simply flying over bodies of water (33%) (Davis, 2019). While the fear is very real for those that experience flight anxiety, the probability of actually becoming a participant in a plane crash is slim. With recent iPhone applications like "Am I Going Down?," where users can check their flight path, type of aircraft, and airline to calculate the probability of crashing, you have to culminate 67,833 years of flying before you reach near certainty of crashing (99%) (Lane, 2015). But, the notion of "it only takes one crash if I'm on the plane" overwhelms the psyche and takes over all logic. Additionally, flight anxiety can skew the perceptions of how safe (or unsafe) air travel really is (Harvell-Bowman & Panetti, 2016). This perception is mediated through self-esteem and pre- and postflight anxiety. Terror Management Theory (TMT), a theory about the unrest that occurs when individuals want to live but know they will die, can help us understand how we psychologically process flight anxiety.

WHAT IS FLIGHT ANXIETY?

There are many different perspectives on flight anxiety and consequently many different definitions. A common measure of flight anxiety is the Flight Anxiety Situations Questionnaire (FASQ). This questionnaire includes three subscales: (1) anticipatory flight anxiety scale—fourteen items related to anxiety regarding anticipating flight, (2) in-flight anxiety scale—eleven items measuring anxiety experienced during a flight, and (3) general flight anxiety scale—seven items investigating anxiety caused in connection with airplanes in general (Nousi, Van Gerwen, & Spinhoven, 2008). Therefore, flight anxiety is a situational phobia, meaning the anxiety is produced by a particular object or situation causing intense anxiety (Mestre et al., 2017). This anxiety often manifests in physiological, psychological, and behavioral reactions (APA, 2013). A fear of loss of control and a need to be in control are key determinants of this anxiety (Van Gerwen et al., 1997; Wilhelm & Roth, 1997). As with other phobias, fear of flying can range from an uncomfortable feeling all the way to an incapacitating phobia where it affects everyday life (Bor, 2007; Van Gerwen, Diekstra, Arondeus, & Wolfger, 2004). Fear of flying is extremely complex psychologically with multiple dimensions (Oakes & Bor, 2010). Both the FASQ and the Flight Anxiety Modality Questionnaire (FAM) are the two primary measures that successfully tap into the nature of flight anxiety.

The FASQ includes thirty-two questions on a five-point scale: 1 = no anxiety to 5 = overwhelming anxiety (see table 1.1) (Van Gerwen, Spinhoven, Van Dick, & Diekstra, 1999). This measure assesses anxiety related to flying, but in various flying situations (e.g., getting ready for a flight, during a flight, during turbulence, etc.).

Complementary to the FASQ, the FAM encompasses eighteen questions on a five-point scale (1 = not at all to 5 = very intensely) and measures physical symptoms and the presence of distressing cognitions (Van Gerwen et al., 1999). The FAM includes two subscales: (1) somatic modality—the physical symptoms one feels with flight anxiety—and (2) cognitive modality—measuring distressing cognitions (see table 1.2; Nousi et al., 2008). Together,

Table 1.1 Flight Anxiety Situations Questionnaire

General Flight Anxiety
1. You see an airplane.
2. You hear the sounds of planes.
3. You read a report about a flight.
4. You bring someone to the airport.
12. You see planes taking off and landing.
Anticipatory Flight Anxiety
9. You enter the departure hall.
11. You are waiting for the boarding call.
15. You are going through the security check.
16. You are going through the gate.
8. You are on the way to the airport.
14. You are walking in the direction of the gate.
10. You are going through customs for a passport check.
7. You buy a ticket.
17. You enter the flight cabin.
18. The doors are being closed.
6. You decide to take a plane.
In-Flight Anxiety
24. The plane banks left or right.
25. The wings of the plane are moving, shaking.
28. The plane starts the descent.
30. You are shaken.
31. The sound of the engine gets louder again.
27. The sound of the engines decreases.
29. Air turbulence is announced.
23. You hear some noises during the flight.
22. You are pushed back into your seat.
32. The landing is announced.
21. The engines give full power before takeoff.
26. The cockpit informs you of the actual altitude or flight level.

Source: As cited in Faraci, Triscari, D'Angelo, & Urso (2011).

these two measures give a well-rounded view of one's flight anxiety and the severity of it.

In industrialized countries, roughly 40 percent of those populations fear flying (Ekeberg, Fauske, & Berg-Hansen, 2014; Mülberger, Weik, Pauli, & Wiedemann, 2006). This is your average fear of flying—producing anxiety, but not particularly life-altering. However, in that same population, 20 percent suffer from an extreme fear of flying, termed "aviophobia" (Ekeberg et al., 2014; Mülberger et al., 2006). Aviophobia is a debilitating disorder that requires people that have the disorder to either be heavily medicated while flying or simply avoid flying altogether (Busscher & Spinhoven, 2017; Kaaij, Garnefski, & Van Gerwen, 2003). This extreme form of flight anxiety is defined by the American Psychiatric Association (2013), where certain

Table 1.2 Flight Anxiety Modality Questionnaire

Somatic Modality
13. I am short of breath.
14. I have the feeling that I am going to choke.
3. I feel pain in the region of my chest.
18. I think that I will faint from fear.
11. I feel dizzy or I have the feeling that I am going to faint.
12. My limbs are tense and cramped, so I feel the urge to move or walk.
15. I have a dry mouth.
17. I feel suddenly warm or cold.
1. I notice numbness in my limbs.
7. The tension makes me clumsy and things fall out of my hands.
Cognitive Modality
9. I attend to every sound or movement of the plane and wonder whether everything is fine.
10. I continuously pay attention to the faces and behavior of the cabin crew.
2. I have a fear of dying.
6. The idea that something will go wrong is constantly in my mind.
8. I can't concentrate because I am preoccupied with thoughts about horrible flight situations.
16. I think the particular plane I am on will crash.
4. I can't tell what is going to happen and that makes me feel very anxious.

Source: As cited in Faraci, Triscari, D'Angelo, & Urso (2011).

characteristics must be present for a diagnosis of aviophobia. In order to be clinically diagnosed with this condition, you must inhabit the following, as outlined in Laker (2012):

1. Exposure to the phobic stimulus produces an immediate anxiety response
2. Response may take the form of a panic attack, even though it is viewed by the sufferer as unreasonable
3. Stimulus is avoided, but met with dread when necessary
4. The avoidance, fear, or anxious anticipation of encounters with the stimulus interferes with everyday life
5. For minors, symptoms must be present for six months
6. There is no other explanation for the anxiety (e.g., OCD, PTSD, social phobia, etc.)

While we do have basis for clinical diagnosis, aviophobia often results from other phobias such as claustrophobia (fear of enclosed spaces), enochlophobia (fear of crowds), acrophobia (fear of heights), and a fear of hijacking or terrorism (Crowley, 2017; Carbonell, 2019; Smith, 2019). While psychology does provide a basis for these fears, a look into the history of this anxiety among aviators as well as sampling some recent plane crashes (and the media that covered them) can provide some insight into why flight anxiety has always been problematic.

HISTORY OF FLIGHT ANXIETY

As early as World War I, military pilots and crew, over time, became quite reluctant to fly, citing insomnia and gastric issues (Laker, 2012). But, at this time, doctors did not have a name for this condition. The condition was later termed "aero-neurosis" due to its somatic nature (Anderson, 1919; Oakes & Bor, 2010). Even though this condition now had a name, it was often attributed to personal temperament, a nervous instability, or even a condition of family history (Laker, 2012). Interest in what we now term "flight anxiety" died down post-World War I, but quickly picked up again with the start of World War II and the increase in usage of airplanes once again (Oakes & Bor, 2010).

In the 1950s, the development of psychotherapy offered a new perspective on this disorder. Sigmund Freud and Carl Jung led this conversation by examining symbols and unconscious processes (Bond, 1952; Oaks & Bor, 2010). Additionally, Freud and Jung argued that love and fear of flying were closely related (Bond, 1952; Oaks & Bor, 2010), providing further guidance into the psychological aspects of this disorder. These perspectives laid the groundwork for what is eventually termed "aviophobia" by the psychological community (Laker, 2012). And, this is how aviophobia is addressed today (Oakes & Bor, 2010). But, who is to blame for this uprising in flight anxiety?

The media and the twenty-four-hour news cycle seem an easy target for the blame of flight anxiety, but perhaps there is more underlying the easy blame. There is empirical research to support that news sources do have a hand in making a more anxious flying public. Seeing images of plane crashes on television, newspapers, or social media adds to this, especially the recent heavy coverage of crashes/missing planes like MH370 (see chapter 6) and MH17 (Cowly, 2017; Carbonell, 2019). But the media should not only be taking the blame. Increased airport security measures such as X-ray scanners and body searches also add to this anxiety (Cowly, 2017). Not surprisingly, past bad experiences, such as turbulence and various air incidents, can also add to the anxiety one feels toward flying (Cowley, 2017; Carbonell, 2019). Last, the mere aspect of having a lack of control while flying is enough to evoke anxiety for some (Ducharme, 2018; Smith, 2019).

With the increase in low-budget airlines such as Frontier and Spirit, air flight is no longer just for the wealthy and middle class. With more options comes an increase in the number of airplanes in the air. For instance, in June 2019 there were 76.8 million passengers on U.S. airlines that month. Air traffic controllers are responsible for guiding all of those passengers to a safe ending (BTS.gov, 2019)—a job not for the faint of heart. In fact, Forbes rated air traffic control as the world's most stressful jobs (Robson, 2020). The more airplanes that are in the air, the more possibility of something going wrong with those airplanes. And, thanks to the twenty-four-hour news cycle, we hear about airplane incidents often. For instance, in 2018, fourteen commercial air incidents occurred. Of those, ten of the incidents had some or all casualties. While only two of these occurred in America (Southwest Flight 1380—suffering a rare engine failure during cruising altitude—and the Horizon Air Q400 hijacking), the media still covered many of the largest casualties, reminding Americans of the reality of plane crashes. There were several crashes covered by the media in 2018 alone, some that were even covered live. But, not all plane crashes are created equal. There are some crashes the media grabs ahold of and dives into, leaving the public psychologically vulnerable.

When considering recent air crashes, a few notable ones come to mind that have the potential to leave a lasting effect on the psyche. In the instance of Iran Aseman Airlines Flight 3704, doubt in the cause of the crash could have caused increased anxiety and media coverage. This Iranian flight, domestic from Tehran to Yasuj, crashed into Mount Dena in the Zagros Mountains in Isfahan Province, causing everybody on board to perish (Selk, 2018). The official cause of the crash was due to icing conditions; however, much of the media focused on the secrecy of Iran's investigation of the crash (Selk, 2018). The BBC capitalized on this uncertainty by heavily focusing on the secrecy, casting further doubt in flyers all over the world.

The idea of who is to blame for a crash is the cause for much anxiety among the flying public. For instance, US-Bangla Airlines Flight 211, an international flight from Dhaka, Bangladesh, to Kathmandu, Nepal, crashed on landing and fifty-one of the seventy-one passengers perished, leaving the survivors badly burned (Wrigley, 2019). The investigation claimed pilot error as the cause with a loss of situational awareness; however, some argue that air traffic control was to blame (Wrigley, 2019). In an article by *the New York Times*, it is posited that the pilot had an emotional breakdown leading to the crash (Sharma, 2019). However, sometimes simply the facts of a crash can be most terrifying, as was the case with Southwest Flight 1380.

Southwest Flight 1380 was heavily covered by the media not only because it was an American flight but because during a sudden decompressurization, a passenger was partially ejected and later died—a rarity even among the most gruesome of crashes (Hoopfer, 2018). This flight, originating at LaGuardia in New York, was headed to Love Field in Dallas, Texas, but had an engine malfunction midflight, also a rarity (Hoopfer, 2018). Later, the National Transportation and Safety Board (NTSB) revealed the piece of the engine that malfunctioned was not subject to certification processes, so the tiny tears in the engine part were missed (Hoopfer, 2018). While Southwest 1380 features several rare events, these events most likely were not in the realm of possibility for passengers and not something commonly worried about among flyers. But, a maintenance error such as the one suffered by flight 1380 breeds mistrust among the flying public and panic can ensue—in this case, there was much talk about whether sitting next to a window was even safe anymore.

The twenty-four-hour news cycle has allowed us to digest plane crash news in unhealthy ways. Specifically, when an air emergency occurs, it can be viewed in real time as was the case with the Horizon Air Q400 incident involving a hijacked aircraft. The regional jet was stolen by a Horizon Air Ground Service Agent with no pilot experience, taking off from Seattle-Tacoma International Airport (Josephs, 2018). The hijacker intentionally crashed the plane on Ketron Island in Puget Sound, all of it covered live by every major American news organization. This type of live coverage of air incidents is not new but can only add to anxiety with the uncertainty of what one might see on live television. Reporting on a crash is scary, but watching the crash live can be absolutely terrifying—anything could happen with live television.

While individual crashes can be disturbing, when a specific aircraft model has problems, the distrust lies in the very making of the aircraft, and the distrust can wreak havoc on the psyche. Lion Air Flight 610 was the first flight to suggest there may be issues with the Boeing 737-MAX aircraft and was of deep interest for Americans. This domestic flight originated from Soekarno-Hatta International Airport in Jakarta to Depati Amir Airport in Pangkal Pinang and crashed twelve minutes after takeoff in the Java Sea (Limer, 2019). The Lion Air Flight 610 crash was the first of two crashes that led to the Boeing 737-MAX aircraft being grounded worldwide, leading to worldwide media coverage.

During 2019, the public was bombarded with constant media coverage of the Boeing 737-MAX crisis. This aircraft is a narrow-body plane and is the fourth generation of the 737. The MAX's first flight was in 2016, but soon thereafter some serious problems began to emerge. First, the Lion Air Flight 610 crashed in 2018. While that crash was being investigated, Ethiopian Airlines Flight 302 (another 737-MAX aircraft) crashed a short few months later. Shortly after the Ethiopian crash, the jets were finally grounded around the world indefinitely (Josephs, 2019), and have recently begun flying again in December 2020.

There was constant media coverage of the 737-MAX issues, canceled flights, and blame placed on Boeing. Both Boeing and the Federal Aviation

Administration (FAA) have faced multiple investigations into their status quos, and the credibility of Boeing's attention to safety has been nearly ruined (Josephs, 2019). These issues have made the public really question Boeing's care for their safety, with good reason, and many airlines too. Because the MAX aircraft were grounded indefinitely, many airlines were turning to Boeing's competitors for reliable aircraft, most notably Boeing's European rival, Airbus. For instance, during the crisis United Airlines purchased twenty Airbus 319s versus purchasing Boeing aircraft (Valinsky, 2019). But, it is not only the American Airlines showing Boeing the door. In 2019, a Saudi budget airline purchased thirty Airbus aircraft replacing a $6 billion agreement they had with Boeing for the 737-MAX (Batrawy, 2019). The public is also not pleased with Boeing. Because Boeing's response to the Lion and Ethiopian crashes were delayed apologies and confusing messages, the response (or lack thereof) caused people anxiety and mistrust—Boeing seemed to simply not care (Baker, 2019). Boeing ended up firing their CEO and worked closely with the FAA to repair and redeem the 737-MAX to get it ready to fly again. In late 2020, the FAA has cleared the Boeing 737-MAX to fly again with American Airlines having the first flight with the aircraft in mid-December 2020. Airlines like Ryan Air, an Irish budget airline, have begun purchasing the 737-MAX again. But, only time will tell if the public will ever feel comfortable on the 737-MAX. If these kinds of issues are causing most of the regular non-anxious flying public anxiety, you can imagine what those effects might look like with someone who has aviophobia.

FLIGHT ANXIETY *IS* DEATH ANXIETY

At the heart of this anxiety is something that is rarely, if ever, mentioned when discussing aviophobia: a fear of death. While there is a lot of discussion of what contributes to this anxiety, the one linkage is what can happen during a crash—you could die. Because of this, flight anxiety takes on a more personal effect; this type of anxiety is existential.

Flight anxiety and death anxiety are woven together to result in an existential nightmare for passengers who are unable to handle both. There has only been one study to date that investigates this relationship. Harvell and colleagues (Harvell, Stillman, Nisbett, Cranney, & Schow, 2016) argue these two psychological constructs are similar. This study found that not only were most passengers anxious, but of those anxious passengers, most cited their fear of being in a crash and probable death. In fact, one passenger stated, "Ever see *Lost*? Well . . . that," in response to why he/she was anxious to fly. In the first episode of *Lost*, the plane crash featured is violent with bodies being ejected from the plane. Of those survivors, they were stuck on a deserted island that, through the series, became its own version of hell on earth. Additionally, a measure traditionally used to pick up death anxiety, picked the anxiety up among the anxious flying public, more so than those who were not anxious.

Harvell and colleagues (2016) further argue that flight anxiety and death anxiety *do* appear to work the same, producing the same kind of existential defense that is typically seen in research investigating death anxiety. Having this type of anxiety among the flying public has the potential to produce grave consequences. For instance, engaging in risky behavior (Taubman Ben-Ari, 2000; Taubman Ben-Ari, Florian, & Mikulincer, 1999), such as violent acts in airports, or worse, in flight. TMT can help provide some insight into the psychological constructs that might cause these types of behaviors in response to anxiety.

TMT, a theory originating in psychology, examines the psychological effects of pondering one's death. When one begins to ponder death, the anxiety of the impending doom creeps in (Becker, 1974). And, as humans, we will do whatever we can to defend against the uncomfortable feelings of death and attempt to alleviate the anxiety (Pyszczynski et al., 1999). This theory, outlined in chapter 2, is at the heart of understanding why flight anxiety is so troubling and a potentially hazardous characteristic of the flying public.

BOOK PREVIEW

This book is meant to bridge theory and application to discuss the perils of flight anxiety among the flying public. Furthermore, this book offers suggestions to journalists and aviation professionals on how to help curb this anxiety to create a healthier flying public. Chapter 2 will feature an overview of TMT and the relevant research related to death anxiety and flight anxiety in regard to this theory. Specifically, a case is made for how the theory can be a guide to understand the psychological processes of flight anxiety and how flight anxiety and death anxiety have similar effects on the psyche.

Chapter 3 provides an overview of research completed at Las Vegas McCarran International Airport examining flight anxiety and testing the differences with death anxiety. This chapter focuses on the grave implications of this, specifically how this type of anxiety has the potential to psychologically put passengers in a bad place. This chapter argues that this type of anxiety has the potential to manifest itself as unfavorable behaviors such as midair brawls, airport shootings, and extreme discomfort among passengers.

Chapter 4 features plane crash survivor stories. Transcripts of the interviews are analyzed with the theoretical guidance of TMT.

Chapter 5 examines what the media's role is in the flight anxiety discussed in the previous chapters. It features three quantitative empirical studies examining the psychological effects of plane crash media coverage in a lab setting. Implications are discussed in this chapter for both TMT and the relationship between the reporting of plane crash news and the public.

Chapter 6 will examine the special case of Cable News Network's (CNN's) coverage of MH370. There was much discussion about how this particular incident, involving a missing aircraft, was constant. Implications of this will be discussed as well as the larger conversation that occurred as a result of this type of coverage.

Chapter 7 merges the areas of psychology, communication, and public relations to form recommendations for practitioners in the aviation industry as well as journalists on how we as a community can begin to try to help curb some of this anxiety.

The last chapter discusses what the public can do to help curb anxiety, specifically detailing how to handle a lack of control in a situation where death is possible.

Chapter 2

Terror Management Theory

A Brief Background

We are, from a purely biological perspective, simply breathing pieces of defecating meat, no more significant or enduring than a lizard or a potato.

—Sheldon Solomon

TMT, originating in psychology in the late 1980s, was first set forth to answer the question of why people strive for self-esteem (Greenberg, Pyszczynski, & Solomon, 1986). However, the late 1980s is not the first mention of the need for self-esteem. Many scholars before have written on this topic (e.g., Adler, 1930; Horney, 1937; James, 1890; Murphy, 1947; Rogers, 1959). Psychotherapists like Horney (1937) have argued continuously how people attempt to defend and enhance self-esteem (see Greenberg et al., 1986 for full review). TMT was first outlined by Jeff Greenberg, Tom Pyszczynski, and Sheldon Solomon in 1986 and is based heavily on the writings of Ernest Becker (1962, 1974, & 1975). Becker outlines how various theorists across several fields have insights regarding the role of self-esteem in social behavior. Theorists such as Sigmund Freud, Erving Goffman, Karen Horney, Søren Kierkegaard, George Herbert Mead, Friedrich Nietzsche, and Otto Rank, to name a few, have written on this topic (Greenberg et al., 1986).

Becker (1962) argues that self-esteem is a uniquely human quality and exists due to our capabilities of reflexive thought. While advanced thought has allowed us to survive, it also allows us to ponder our existence knowing that death is inevitable and could occur at any moment (Becker, 1962; Smith, 1978). Becker (1973, 1975) further argues that when this occurs, we are paralyzed with terror. Unless we can deny the idea of death, the terror will take over, and we will be unable to function. The ability to ponder death has enabled our cognitive capacities as humans to increase, and we have since developed cultural worldviews (CWVs) that provide us with a sense of order, predictability, meaning, and permanence (Greenberg et al., 1986). These CWVs provide a description for how the world was created, leading to a prescription for maintaining a meaningful and good life with the hope of immortality (Becker, 1973, 1975; Greenberg et al., 1986; Rank, 1950).

The ability to ponder meaningfulness in a larger culture makes humans unique. No other animal can do this. In this sense, humans are *cultural* animals living with a shared symbolic conception of the world that is not only determined by culture but also considered the reality of the individual within that culture. The ability to have a symbolic conception of the world is the basis for how an individual values him or herself; symbolic conception is based on the individual satisfying his or her cultural criteria for being good. Therefore, self-esteem is how an individual views themselves as valuable within his/her culture (Greenberg et al., 1986).

When one does not have the safety of feeling valued in his or her culture, feelings of discomfort and uncertainty can arise. Research has consistently shown that individuals chronically low in self-esteem are prone to anxiety (e.g., French, 1968; Greenberg et al., 1986; Rosenberg, 1965; Rosenberg & Simmons, 1972; Winkler & Myers, 1963). Therefore, self-esteem can serve as an anxiety-buffering construct when two components are present. The first component is a faith in a CWV that portrays life as meaningful, important, and enduring. The second component is a belief that one plays a significant role in that CWV (Greenberg et al., 1986). Threats to self-esteem are simply CWV shortcomings of the self (e.g., not living up to your culture's standards) and events that threaten our CWV by suggesting it is not valid (e.g., 9/11) (Greenberg et al., 1986).

When your CWV is threatened, there is an urgency for maintaining the anxiety-buffer, and consequently defense strategies emerge and are aimed at diffusing the threat at an attempt to repair the damage. This can be done in three ways. The first way is sustaining faith in a CWV. Actions that support this are things such as relying on religious beliefs as a way to restore action or displaying cultural symbols (e.g., American flag, currency, religious symbols) and engaging in cultural rituals (e.g., singing national anthem, going to church, visiting historical monuments) (Greenberg et al., 1986). The second way is defending against the threat. By eliminating the threat, our CWV, and consequently our self-esteem, can remain unharmed. America's 9/11 can be used as an example of one such threat. When 9/11 occurred, it was a direct attack on America's culture and value structure, all while making Americans very aware of the fragility of life as they watched people jump to their deaths from the twin towers. The cultural response to this event, extreme patriotism, was a direct defense of the threat against the American CWV. In fact, the entire country shifted slightly conservative after 9/11 (Nail & McGregor, 2009). The military response also served as a defense against the threat. America immediately engaged in a war with the countries responsible for the 9/11 attacks and vowed to catch and put on trial the individual architects of the event, something that later resulted in the death of Osama Bin Laden. This defense made Americans feel superior and thus feeling restored in their cultural belief system. However, this is not only isolated to America.

The Rwandan Genocide can be used as another example of a CWV threat. Following World War II in Rwanda, the Hutu began to become educated and powerful within the Catholic Church, therefore challenging the historically politically elite Tutsi. From there, the Tutsi did not appreciate the change in status from the Hutu and decided to try for immediate independence from the Hutu by labeling the Tutsis and the Hutus as separate races. When a Hutu subchief was attacked near his home by supporters of a pro-Tutsi group, Hutu activists responded by killing Tutsi, and the genocide began. Many Tutsi attempted to escape, but many were not able to, resulting in thousands of deaths. Once the differences were made salient, violence was the answer to show that one race (i.e., one CWV) was superior to the other.

Defending against threats to one's CWV sets up an *us versus them* mentality. Two studies within the TMT literature explain how this works. Three experiments show that defending one's in-group compensates for the loss of control that occurs when realizing the inescapability of death (Agroskin & Jonas, 2013). When pondering death, people immediately seek to identify with like-minded people and consequently defend any attacks against their CWV (Hohman & Hogg, 2015). Therefore, moving into an *us versus them* mentality is somewhat unavoidable and defending against threats to our CWVs is evolutionary.

The third way to maintain your anxiety-buffer when your CWV is threatened is to maintain a sense of personal value within the CWV. In TMT, self-esteem is entirely a cultural creation. You cannot have a sense of self-worth without meeting the expectations of your CWV. So, self-defining goals are a way to attain and maintain CWV beliefs; they help to secure self-esteem (Greenberg et al., 1986).

One problem that arises from this theory that helps shed light on why flight anxiety, specifically those with aviophobia, can be so problematic is this: "A variety of mental health problems may result from the individual's inability to maintain a cultural anxiety-buffer, because of loss of faith either in one's ability to maintain a valued cultural drama or in the cultural drama itself" (Greenberg et al., 1986, p. 207). Those experiencing aviophobia, a recognized clinical disorder, may not have the ability to buffer traditionally held death anxiety, essentially making this terror worse and thus explaining why those with aviophobia are so hard to treat.

PROXIMAL AND DISTAL DEFENSES

When something in the environment causes existential reminders, people tend to engage in what terror management scholars call *proximal defenses* (see figure 2.1). A proximal defense is an immediate denial of death. People will immediately seek to logically deny their impending doom (e.g., I'm probably not going to die today) (Kosloff, Anderson, Nottbohm, & Hoshiko, 2019). In an airport setting, passengers rely on the statistics that you are much more likely to be in a car accident on the way to the airport instead of being involved in a plane crash (Locsin, 2018). However, once denial has taken place, crash thoughts begin to exit the conscious mind and recede into the unconscious.

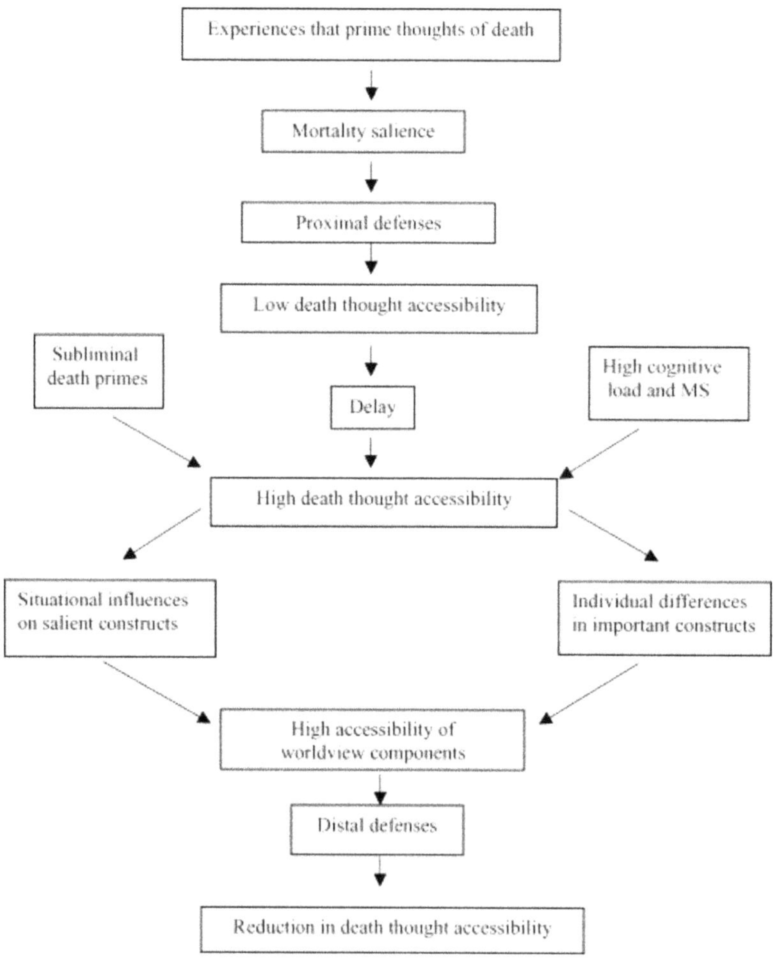

Figure 2.1 Terror Management Model. Note: As cited in Arndt et al., 2005.

When the thoughts of crashing exit the conscious mind, these same people that once exhibited proximal defenses begin to exhibit what terror management scholars term "distal defenses." Distal defenses begin moving around in the unconscious mind and tend to produce responses that are specifically aimed at obtaining self-esteem and maintaining a CWV. Distal defenses tend not to be as logical like proximal defenses, but are deeply personal (Kosloff et al., 2019). Once people engage in these behaviors, the distal defenses reduce the existential angst back to baseline levels (Kosloff et al., 2019). In an airport setting, distal defenses can translate to women having a higher need to use electronic media and eat more unhealthy food (Harvell et al., 2016). Additionally, distal defenses manifest in males as a higher need to gamble (Harvell et al., 2016). The behaviors shown by Harvell and colleagues in 2016 are a direct extension of Taubman Ben-Ari's (2000) assertion that people aware of death often engage in risky behavior.

INITIAL SUPPORT FOR TMT

The first support for TMT emerged in two articles published in 1989 and 1990, respectively. Rosenblatt, Greenberg, Solomon, Pyszczynski, and Lyon (1989) set out to first test the theory through a series of six experiments. These experiments all individually replicated and tested specific tenets of the theory.

The first experiment asked municipal court judges to set bond for a suspected prostitute using the basis of judgments they would normally use to make such judgments. Immediately prior to getting information on the case, mortality was made salient to half of the judges in the study (i.e., the judges pondered their own death). In order to get the judges to ponder their own mortality, open-ended questions were asked concerning their thoughts and feelings about their own death. Results showed that the judges reminded of their own death recommended higher bonds for prostitutes, as predicted. The results of the judge study supported that moral principles were a part of one's CWV and these moral principles protected individuals from the anxiety that occurred from pondering their own death. When these moral views are threatened (i.e., the prostitute), negative reactions toward the transgressor ensued (i.e., higher bonds). By introducing mortality salience (MS), it increased the need for faith in a CWV and thus resulted in a desire to punish the transgressor (in this case, the prostitute).

Because CWVs can vary within individuals from that same culture, the second experiment tested the notion that some may not have overly negative views toward prostitution, thus a premeasure of attitudes toward prostitution was used. This experiment also tested the notion that a negative mood may ensue from pondering death and therefore it could be that mood caused the harsher punishments rather than MS. Results showed that MS did not lead to harsher punishments of *any* target. For instance, there was not an effect on the evaluations of the experimenter, thus suggesting that MS leads only to those threatening a CWV. There was also a lack of effect on the post-manipulation mood measures, further suggesting that MS is causing the harsher punishments. For people with positive views of prostitution, MS did not affect these views because they did not see the prostitute violating any of their important values.

TMT suggests people that uphold the values shared by those believing in a specific CWV will be viewed positively when their views are threatened (Greenberg et al., 1986). The third experiment tested this idea by giving participants the opportunity to determine the reward value for someone that provided police a tip that led to the arrest of a criminal, despite the risk that doing so caused. Results showed that greater rewards were recommended for the hero. These results replicated the effects of the previous experiments that MS affects the punishment of moral transgressors.

Because some of these effects could be explained because of arousal and not just a threat to CWV viewpoints, the fourth experiment included not only setting bond for a prostitute but also rating how much participants liked five pleasant events and five unpleasant events. Also, because MS could solely encourage higher bond values, participants were asked to estimate the value of various consumer products. Results show that self-awareness does not encourage higher bond recommendations, but instead it reduces the harshness of the punishment among those participants that held positive views of prostitution. Additionally, results show that MS does not cause increased monetary estimates on *any* positive or negative stimuli but cause only those stimuli threatening one's CWV. The fifth experiment sought to replicate the fourth experiment while monitoring physiological arousal to better rule out arousal being a factor in MS effects. Results showed no physiological effects while replicating previous effects present. Therefore, physiological arousal appeared to not account for MS effects.

All previous experiments used the same dependent variable: bonds for prostitutes, while knowing it can work for other CWV-threatening topics. Therefore, the sixth experiment wanted to replicate the bond effect through a different MS-inducing mechanism. Instead of the open-ended questions used previously, this experiment used Boyar's (1964) Fear of Death scale to make mortality salient among participants. Results confirm that the MS effects found in experiments 1 to 5 are not simply due to the open-ended questions, but truly caused by people pondering their own death. This initial article provides great evidence for TMT but also makes a call to answer the still unanswered questions regarding the functions of culture, values, and self-esteem that TMT argues must be considered.

Greenberg, Rosenblatt, Veeder, Kirkland, and Lyon (1990) provide the second article that aims to test TMT. The three experiments showcased in this manuscript test the prediction by TMT that when people are reminded of death, attraction to those validating their beliefs are increased, while decreasing it for those that threaten their beliefs.

The first experiment examines the effects of MS on reactions to those with similar and dissimilar religious backgrounds. Results showed that when having Christians think about their own mortality, these thoughts led them to provide more positive interpersonal judgments of fellow Christians and more negative interpersonal judgments of Jews. These findings suggest that these positive reactions to in-groups and negative reactions to out-groups are mediated by the need for these individuals to have for their CWV. But, according to TMT, *any* threat to a CWV should cause these effects, not solely religious beliefs.

TMT argues that MS will increase the similarity-attraction relationship, leading people to have a larger liking for similar people and a much lesser liking for those that are dissimilar. The second experiment tests this argument while also examining individual differences in interpersonal responses to MS because everybody's perspective of their culture and what is important within that culture can differ. Results show that MS causes high authoritarians to derogate those that are dissimilar only when people pondered their own death. Those with authoritarian personality characteristics tend to have a high level of respect for authority, rigid and dogmatic views, and have negative attitudes toward those who are different. Interestingly, this finding was only found among high authoritarians, while low authoritarians showed none of these effects. So, the question then remained if low authoritarians engaged in terror management and if these people were even remotely concerned with their own mortality.

Greenberg and colleagues (1990) offer three explanations as to why MS effects may not be able to be seen among low authoritarians. First, there is a lot of evidence suggesting that death awareness is widespread, even with people that deny it in self-report measures (Alexander, Colley, & Adlerstein, 1957; Greenberg et al., 1990; Templer, 1971). It is possible that the death anxiety of low authoritarians was not being self-reported, despite it being present. Second, powerful effects have been discovered of MS in other studies (Greenberg et al., 1990; Rosenblatt et al., 1989), suggesting authoritarianism not being a problem. Last, because low authoritarians are generally open-minded, MS would not trigger them to act negatively to those that were dissimilar.

The first two experiments in the Greenberg et al. (1990) research as well as the previously discussed Rosenblatt et al. (1989) research argue for indirect validations or threats to CWVs. If effects are present for indirect threats, it would be expected that direct threats would cause an even stronger reaction, something that Experiment 3 examines. Results show that MS continues to encourage positive reactions to people praising their culture and consequently negative reactions to those that criticize their culture. But, the credentials of the interviewee did not alter the effects of MS. So, reactions to the interviewee depended entirely on his/her view of the culture and not his/her group status. This suggests that terror management may play a role in not only the promotion of nationalism and censorship but also the persecution of those that challenge a popular worldview.

The studies initially testing TMT are groundbreaking not only because they provide the initial evidence for TMT but also because they provide psychologists with a solution for why prejudice and hostility toward different others occurs—a potentially costly way of coping with fears and insecurities. Thus, decades of research spun off of these studies investigating a wide array of topics and theoretical extensions.

TMT TODAY

Since the theory's inception, four meta-analyses (i.e., a summary of a group of research studies) have been conducted on the several decades of TMT research in a variety of areas. The first of these emerged in 2010 specifically to examine the strength of MS effects and if these effects were moderated by variations in TMT experiment characteristics. This research suggested that the effects produced in laboratories may be very different from real-world death experiences like terminal illnesses, which is usually met with liberation and growth (Burke, Martens, & Faucher, 2010). Burke and colleagues (2010) called for more research to examine those that experience death in their everyday lives (e.g., morticians, hospice workers, etc.). The second meta-analysis questioned the Burke et al. (2010) findings due to the fear that researcher effect may be causing the MS effects. This research showed this fear as being a real possibility citing experimental procedure and publication bias (Yen & Cheng, 2013). The third meta-analysis emerged around the same time as the previous, except the latter examined MS effects on political attitudes. This research showed that conservative shifting (i.e., all viewpoints, regardless of ideology, shifting conservatively) was a response to existential threat and was likely among conservatives *and* liberals when the cultural climate was conservative (Burke, Kosloff, & Landau, 2013). Right after 9/11, conservatism provided psychological security (Burke et al., 2013). The last and most recent research overview provided analysis of close relationships and MS effects. This meta-analysis showed that close relationships continue to play an important role in buffering death anxiety (Plusnin, Pepping, & Kashima, 2018). The most influential psychological characteristics associated with close relationships that had an effect on MS were attachment, gender, and relationship-contingent self-esteem (Plusnin, Pepping, & Kashima, 2018).

There have also been several books published on TMT. In 2015, the founders of this theory, Sheldon Solomon, Jeff Greenberg, and Tom Pyszczynski, wrote about TMT summarizing the research, but targeting it to a popular audience. In 2016, Lindsey Harvell and Gwendelyn Nisbett published an edited volume featuring interdisciplinary research on TMT and argued the wide range and applicability the theory has in multiple disciplines. In 2019, Clay Routledge and Matthew Vess published a similar book with additional interdisciplinary research, a handbook of recent TMT interdisciplinary research. In 2020, Ken Vail and Clay Routledge published an edited volume on existentialism, religion, and spirituality. The current book will be the next in line offering insights into the applicability of TMT in the aviation industry.

In the past year, much of TMT research is focused around mindfulness and meditation practices. The first study showed there were less proximal (i.e., immediate) responses with mindfulness and mind-wandering when compared to a worry group, but no effects were found for distal (i.e., delayed response) outcomes (Schultz & Arnau, 2019). This line of research further suggests that mindfulness may effectively buffer the negative affect associated with MS, however, simply letting the mind wander also produces these effects (Schultz & Arnau, 2019). Research in mindfulness has also shown that a "mindfulness of death" can have a positive psychological impact and can be used to induce MS (Moon, 2019). Specific psychological changes that occur were shown to increase pro-social attitudes which can emphasize ethics and morality and can also emphasize the intrinsic value of life due to the ties to CWV and self-esteem (Moon, 2019). Last, recent research has shown that death thought accessibility (i.e., how aware you are of thoughts of death) was a mediator regarding the effect of MS on worldview defense without meditation (Park & Pyszczynski, 2019). But, when meditation was added, this mediation disappeared (Park & Pyszczynski, 2019). This suggests some subtle differences in mindfulness research and one that will no doubt continue to be worked out in the literature.

The remaining recent literature is centered around the original tenets of TMT. The largest set features three studies examining CWVs. Naveh-Kedem and Sverdlik (2019) argue that existential threats cause value change and examined this through the context of armed conflicts in Israel. This study continues with the notion that armed conflicts are real-life examples of existential threats and existential threat moderates the effects on universalism. In fact, this research showed that the very manipulation of MS increases the importance of benevolence (Naveh-Kedem & Sverdlik, 2019). Similar to this research is one that examines whether MS and tolerance salience influences the endorsement of anti-Islamic attitudes in American politics and political orientation. Specifically, when neutral values were present, individuals aware of their death more strongly endorsed anti-Islamic statements of a congressman when compared to individuals not aware of their death (Vail, Courtney, & Arndt, 2019). However, when tolerance values were present, those individuals aware of their own death were more accepting of those same anti-Islamic statements. No effects for political orientation were found (Vail et al., 2019). Last, Schindler and colleagues (2019) showed that individuals aware of their own death showed less dishonest behavior and more specifically, showed honest behavior when given an incentive to cheat.

Two recent research studies examine the last two tenets of the theory: self-esteem and MS. Gerber and Anaki (2019) posited that self-esteem can lead to the devaluation of others and that perhaps self-compassion is a more inclusive construct than self-esteem. Results of this research showed that self-compassion was not associated with the avoidance of abstract threats but associated with concrete threats. This suggests the potential for self-compassion to help with trauma and even perhaps the prevention of Post-Traumatic Stress Disorder (Gerber & Anaki, 2019). Recent studies have also shown that people reading articles stating that certain animals (in this study's context, dolphins) were smarter than humans had higher levels of death-related thoughts (Soenke, Cohen, Greenberg, & Lifshin, 2018), suggesting that these people were threatened by what they were reading.

While the current research has gone in various directions, this book suggests that MS may be psychologically similar to another construct: flight anxiety. And, if this is the case, then airports and airlines should be deeply concerned about the psychological well-being of their passengers. But, how is flight anxiety similar to MS?

THE SIMILARITIES BETWEEN MORTALITY SALIENCE AND FLIGHT ANXIETY

Even if you are not an anxious flyer, getting ready for a flight and the airport processes immediately preceding your flight can be stressful to even the calmest of flyers. In addition to that stress, airports are full of reminders of death. First, security. As you wait in an often-long line, and as you go through that line, there is a reminder of why there are such strict security policies at airports (either consciously or unconsciously). You might be reminded of 9/11 and what these planes can be used for—not the most pleasant thought as you board one of these potential flying coffins. Second, once you have boarded the airplane, you hear a safety message: a message that reminds you what to do in case of an emergency in flight. Safety messages are the most overt death reminders you will encounter on an airplane, next to actually being in an emergency. Interestingly, the most common reaction of passengers is not to listen to these messages.

There is only one study to date that holds the first empirical evidence of the link between the fear associated with the topic of death and the fear of events that potentially lead to death. Outlined by Lancaster, Bowman, and Harvell (2016), this study argued that if people are primed to think about death via a fear appeal (e.g., being told they will die if the airplane they are on crashes), but also told that if they pay attention to the safety message, they could potentially save themselves, that those people would be most likely to pay attention to the safety demonstration video. Interestingly, the results of this research show that airline passengers might not pay attention to the videos regardless of how much information they are given about how likely they are to die in a crash but how there is something they can do about it (i.e., become familiar with the safety procedures set forth in the safety demonstration videos). In fact, most participants in the Lancaster et al. study were unable to recall any of the steps outlined in the video. This suggests an unconscious reaction to exposure to death reminders, a proximal defense. Further, by pushing the message away (i.e., not paying attention and not recalling safety procedures), this action can be directly translated to death denial.

Another study that directly suggests a psychological similarity between flight anxiety and death anxiety is set forth in the research conducted by Harvell and colleagues (2016) with passengers at Las Vegas McCarran International Airport (LAS) in Las Vegas, Nevada. This study shows that people are anxious to fly because they fear something bad will happen (i.e., death). A qualitative analysis of writings from passengers showed that passenger anxieties at LAS were tied to potential crashes, and consequently these passengers were very anxious and death aware, which puts the flying public in a rather grave psychological state.

Chapter 3

Similarities between Flight Anxiety and Death Anxiety

A pilot who says he has never been frightened in an airplane is, I'm afraid, lying.

—Louise Thaden

My research team and I arrived at LAS on a cool spring day, March 7, 2014, greeted by the LAS public affairs team. Our goal that day was a lofty one—to speak to as many passengers at as many gates and terminals as possible to assess flight anxiety. As existential psychologists, we were interested in how the process of getting ready for a flight and being at the airport affects flight anxiety as well as the psychological similarities to death anxiety. Unaware to researchers at the time, this data would be a baseline of flight anxiety prior to a string of air disasters. We just happened to be at LAS the day prior to Malaysia Airlines Flight 370 going missing, and a variety of other air disasters that occurred in the months and years that followed (e.g., MH17, Germanwings 9525, etc.).

LAS is different from other American airports. Las Vegas is known for gambling, something the airport prominently features throughout LAS, offering passengers a unique airport experience. Additionally, like most airports, there are a variety of consumerism options at LAS, from food to low-end goods to luxury items. Because LAS had some characteristics of most U.S. airports, it also offered a gambling option; thus this airport was an ideal place to study flight anxiety and its effects on consumerism. We were able to talk to passengers in every terminal, including international passengers. And, for American passengers, every geographic location was represented.

Flying is scary, regardless of whether you are a frequent flyer or not. And, we know that eventually individuals can snap under stress. For passengers, these snaps can happen in an airport, or even worse, on a plane. The flying public are anxious to fly because of the potential *bad* things that could happen, with the worst, of course, being crashing. Graduate students analyzed paragraphs the passengers wrote about regarding their anxieties about flight. Most of the accounts focused on crashing, or things that can lead to a crash, such as a malfunctioning airplane. Terrorism was a concern as well as some being concerned about the people sitting next to them. And, only a handful of passengers said they lacked flight anxieties. If this question was asked today, almost six years later, I suspect being shot down, going missing, or the pilot's mental health may be adding to these anxieties.

The LAS data suggests that passengers *are* afraid of dying due to a crash. In fact, measures that are used to pick up death anxiety were used with passengers in this study and those with flight anxiety showed relatively high levels of death anxiety. The fact is, dying is at the root of flight anxiety. The LAS study was the first research to suggest that flight anxiety and death anxiety are psychologically similar. So, given that assumption, keeping airports and airplanes safe with an anxious public becomes much more difficult.

THE CONSEQUENCES OF FLIGHT ANXIETY

As air travel has continued to increase over the decades, so has general anxiety. In 2018, 6.8 million American adults suffered from Generalized Anxiety Disorder, 6 million American adults suffered from a panic disorder, and a staggering 15 million American adults suffered from a social anxiety disorder (Anxiety and Depression Association of America, 2018). Additionally, 19 million American adults suffered from specific phobias, such as aviophobia, a fear of flying (Anxiety and Depression Association of America, 2018). This suggests, much like what we found at LAS, that, in general, the flying public is quite anxious. When people have anxiety, it can be accompanied by other disorders, making the anxiety symptoms worse in many cases and hard to treat (Anxiety and Depression Association of America, 2018). In fact, aviophobia can often be linked to other primary causes of anxiety such as the fear of enclosed spaces (claustrophobia), a fear of crowds (agoraphobia), a fear of heights (acrophobia), and even the anxiety of not being in control (N.A., 2019). With all of these possibilities for anxiety, when passengers get stressed, certain unsavory behaviors can manifest as a result of this anxiety.

With the increase in flights come increases in delays. And, when there are delays, passengers get angry. But, is it getting worse? Some would suggest so. In 2017, there was 1 unruly passenger incident for every 1,053 flights (IATA, 2019). And, in the ten years prior to that, there were over 66,000 incidents (IATA, 2019). These incidents undoubtedly cause more anxiety by causing further delays and diversions. However, the problem may be much worse than what is being reported by the International Air Transport Association (IATA), because not all airlines in the world are members of IATA, and this organization only reports what members report (Street, 2019). The FAA tallies their own data on unruly passengers, and it shows widely ranging numbers (see table 3.1). From 1995 to 2019, the numbers range anywhere on a low end of 87 incidents a year to a high end of 310 incidents a year. There are not really any patterns, either. The highest, 310 incidents, were in 2004 with the second highest number of incidents, 305, being in 2001. This level of incidents would be somewhat expected with the anxiety that may have been caused post-9/11. However, the numbers were on the decline in 2018.

Some of these incidents may not only be related to anxiety. And, how passengers handle varying levels of anxiety can lead to violent behavior in the

Table 3.1 FAA Unruly Passengers Count

"Unruly Passengers"	
Calendar Years 1995–2019	
Year	*Total*
2019	87 as of December 13, 2019
2018	153
2017	91
2016	102
2015	105
2014	147
2013	149
2012	183
2011	155
2010	128
2009	139
2008	124
2007	153
2006	137
2005	205
2004	310
2003	286
2002	279
2001	305
2000	255
1999	226
1998	204
1997	237
1996	184
1995	146

Source: As cited from https://www.faa.gov/data_research/passengers_cargo/unruly_passengers/.

air (Mous & Thomas, 2001). Passengers with preexisting mental health issues and phobias related to air travel are at higher risk for an air rage incident. For instance, in 2018, an Aeroflot passenger violently attacked a flight attendant over a missing cell phone that was in his possession the entire time. In that same year, a United Express passenger flying in first class had an outburst that caused her to attempt to open the emergency door while yelling, "I am God!" And, while not all of these incidents are violent, some can be quite grotesque. For instance, in 2018, a Frontier Airlines passenger grabbed two women and urinated on the seat directly in front of them (Fox News, 2018). So, what else besides flight anxiety could be causing this aggressive behavior? For one, people with thicker superior-frontal cortexes are more likely in general to exhibit aggressive behavior (Zhu et al., 2020). In fact, research has shown that when combined with traits such as high negative affect and neuroticism, these individuals can exhibit more aggression (Zhu et al., 2020). Other types of anxieties could lead some people to interpret ambiguous behavior of others (e.g., flight attendants or other passengers) as hostile, termed the "Hostile Attribution Bias" (Klein Truente, Bogaetrts, & Veling, 2019). Aggression and hostility among certain individuals have been consistently seen across a diverse group of populations. But, passengers without any preexisting conditions can also be at risk. Some have even cited hypoxia and/or dehydration leading to some of these unruly behaviors (Street, 2019). But the cause of air rage should not lie solely on the passenger; the airlines also have their role in this aggression.

While commercial airline passengers are generally happy with their overall flying experience (Schaper, 2017), they seem to be increasingly unhappy with legroom and seat width while on the aircraft (Mous & Thomas, 2001; Paul, 2018; Schaper, 2017; Spinks, 2018a). As passengers unwillingly have to encroach on others' space, tensions can arise. Adding to these tensions is the fact that if a passenger finds himself/herself in one of these situations, he/she cannot simply walk away—these passengers are stuck. Not to mention, these violent situations could potentially be fueled by alcohol. In fact, alcohol is the primary fuel for air rage (Mous & Thomas, 2001). The problem is then put back on the airports and airlines: Why not just stop serving alcohol? Because it generates a large portion of revenue for airlines and airports (Spinks, 2018b). And, while flight attendants and airports do refuse alcohol to those passengers who clearly have had enough, the refusal of alcohol often initiates the violent behavior, putting us back at square one (Mous & Thomas, 2001). Passengers have not been allowed to smoke on planes since 1990 (Reed, 2015). And, a fair amount of research has suggested that when nicotine-addicted passengers go without nicotine on longer flights, levels of stress increase (Mous & Thomas, 2001). In addition to alcohol and nicotine withdrawal symptoms, passengers can also be under the influence of illegal drugs through ingesting them or transportation of them inside their bodies (Department of Homeland Security, 2017). In 2019, U.S. Customs and Border Patrol apprehended 2,549 lbs of Fentanyl, 5,427 lbs of heroin, 68,585 lbs of methamphetamine, 89,207 lbs of cocaine, and an impressive 289,529 lbs of marijuana (Customs and Border Patrol, 2019).

WHAT CAN AIRPORTS AND AIRLINES DO TO HELP?

Before passengers even arrive at the airport, they are stressed with worries like getting stuck on the way to the airport, missing the boarding time, delays, and needing to pay extra for baggage (Priority Pass, 2019). And then once arriving at the airport, passengers are plagued with anxiety related to checking in and security. While moving walkways can help passengers get from place to place quick and efficiently, these walkways are often narrow and do not promote enough room for varying speeds of movement with bags. Many airports are old and outdated. Oftentimes, these airports would require a major overhaul to put in passenger comforts like moving walkways.

Since 2008, U.S. airports have spent $54 billion for capital improvement projects and globally, $385 billion for airport improvement projects (Sharkey, 2015). Researchers have recently called on airports to adopt the concept of flexibility. The concept of flexibility is used in design to explain how one might change the mode of operation or the attribute of a system to meet the demands of changing needs (Chant, 2015; Edwards, 2005; Shuchi, 2016). For airports, this translates to an infrastructure being able to adapt to future needs with minimal investment (Shuchi, Drogemuller, & Buys, 2017). Elements such as connected buildings and shared spaces, such as waiting areas in front of gates, make changes to that space in the future much easier (de Neufville & Odoni, 2003). Having a flexible concept in mind during airport design could help alleviate anxiety through ease of passenger travel not only through the airport but also during times of renovation.

Engineers have called on future airport designs to encompass (1) more comfortable handling of passengers, (2) capacity *and* qualitative increases, and (3) using clean energy products (Medvedev, Alomar, & Augustyn, 2017). Most argue that airport design needs to incorporate large passenger capacity with a high level of passenger comfort—for everybody, not just those with elite club memberships (Medvedev et al., 2017). So, what does a flexible concept design look like in today's world? It looks like Singapore Changi Airport (SIN)—an airport so nice, and so comfortable, that people beg for long layovers here.

SINGAPORE CHANGI AIRPORT

The newly designed SIN opened its new attractions in April 2019. This new masterfully designed airport has the capability of handling around twenty million passengers (Beckerling, 1997). And, passengers have repeatedly ranked this airport as one of the most efficient and inviting airports in the world (Weathersby, 2003). Terminal 1 features a rooftop swimming pool and hot tub as well as a cactus garden (Cartledge, 2016). Terminal 2 features a sunflower garden that doubles as a viewing terrace, giving passengers an opportunity for plane spotting and fresh tropical air during a layover (Cartledge, 2016). Terminal 3 features a roof made up of computer-controlled reflectors that allow natural light in while keeping the tropical heat out (Cartledge, 2016). While all of the terminals have received upgrades, it is Terminal 2 that received the largest overhaul that took approximately five years to complete. The entire airport features butterfly gardens, paint areas for kids, PlayStation/Xbox consoles, music corners, and television lounges (Cartledge, 2016; Sharkey, 2015).

Terminal 2 is essentially what sealed the deal for SIN to become the world's best airport. The terminal features a giant 1,460,662 square feet mall that is disguised by a large atrium garden, complete with a 131 foot waterfall with large canyons and a valley (Post, 2019). The waterfall is often used for 360-degree sound and light shows for passengers as they pass through the terminal. The retail spaces are completely hidden in a five-level forest. The forest features more than 2,000 trees, palms, and over 100,000 shrubs, all originating from Australia, China, Malaysia, Spain, Thailand, and the United States (Post, 2019). The waterfall can process an impressive 100,000 gallons of water per minute at its maximum during heavy rainfall—something that can occur frequently in Singapore (Correa, 2019). If this was not enough, the terminal also features a hotel and a twenty-four-hour movie theatre. However, the terminals are not the only thing that will impress you; getting around SIN is a comfortable and awe-inspiring adventure as well. The transit station leading to the airport shares the same features as Terminal 2—a three-story atria which allows daylight to flood what would normally be dark, interior spaces (Weathersby, 2003).

The overall goal for SIN was to bring in as much light as possible (Correa, 2019). It has been stated in a travel review, "For the 85 million people estimated to visit each year, they won't just go to travel. They'll go to walk through the gardens, stand by the waterfall, and look up at the sky" (Correa, 2019). With this perspective, you cannot help but think that flight anxiety would be naturally reduced because the airport is a comforting place—the light, the trees, and all of it. In fact, research suggests that being connected to nature has the ability to lower anxiety.

When we partake in nature-based experiences, we experience boosts in psychological well-being and overall mental health (Röderer & Cervinka, 2012). An effect that some might argue is stronger than physical activity alone (Mitchell, 2013). At the end of the day, as we become more connected to nature, our anxiety levels drop. A recent study showed that individuals experiencing nature stated this experience gave them the opportunity to take time from their days to relax and have fun (Martyn & Brymer, 2016). While SIN is truly amazing in its design, American airports still have a long way to go to reach this point, but the amenities in American airports *are* getting better (Sharkey, 2015). While SIN is far away from American travelers, there is an airport within America that has undergone extreme renovations with passenger comfort in mind.

LOUIS ARMSTRONG NEW ORLEANS INTERNATIONAL AIRPORT

For years, the Louis Armstrong New Orleans International Airport (MSY) was dreaded by passengers. Not only was the airport old and run-down, but it was also often cramped and crowded—a quality that reached unbearable during Mardi Gras. In November 2019, MSY unveiled their new $826 million new terminal featuring open air, tall ceilings, and wide-open spaces (Adelson, Simerman, & Calder, 2019). While the old airport featured generic food chains, the new MSY invested $10 million to showcase the taste and look of New Orleans throughout the airport (Ahmad, 2014). Even the author of this book experienced the New Orleans flair in the United Club on the club's opening day in late February 2020. The restaurants in the airport are New Orleans–themed and reflect New Orleans pricing, rather than the normal inflated airport pricing. Additionally, the stores and restaurants have different store hours to better fit the needs of New Orleans passengers (Ahmad, 2014).

The new terminal features a consolidated (and centralized) security screening checkpoint and a roomy airline check-in and baggage claim area (Adelson et al., 2019). In fact, the light and architecture in the new MSY have been described as downright lovely in airport reviews (Adelson et al., 2019). The new MSY design has the potential to reduce anxiety, but in this airport's case, not everybody has been pleased. The reviews of the opening were mixed, citing major organizational challenges within management. So, even when airports are designed with the best intentions of flexibility, things can still go wrong. And, anxiety may still be present or may be even worse. For instance, getting to the new MSY is a challenge. While there are plans to connect a highway to the terminal, the current road is riddled with potholes and stoplights (Leigh, 2019). Other complaints are that while the security screening process is consolidated, the one large screening area can create long lines. Additionally, rental cars are located on the other side of the airfield leaving passengers with quite the commute (Leigh, 2019). So, while airport designers can focus heavily on passenger comfort when designing new spaces, in the case of MSY, it appears that airport management is the source of the anxiety.

THE IMPORTANCE OF AIRPORT MANAGEMENT

Airport design may not be the only way airports can help curb anxiety. Airport management may also play a role. For instance, while many airlines now offer online check-in services, passengers are often still required to drop bags off in lines that can be quite long in addition to security lines having the potential to be long and cumbersome, making passengers anxious and uncomfortable before they even enter the departure hall.

With the potential of a psychologically unhealthy flying public, myself and colleague, Dr. Tatjana Hocke-Mirzashvilli, took a look at how the messaging of airport management could play a role. Risk perception research suggests that a number of factors influence how a risk is perceived (Ferrer & Klein, 2015). These factors include control, experience, knowledge, and familiarity with the risk. Flying is often *perceived* as riskier than traveling by car, something we know is simply not true. This incorrect judgment of risk can be attributed to a lack of control when flying and less overall knowledge and experience with flight. To assess the connection between risk perception and flight anxiety, Hocke-Mirzashvilli and myself sought to capture perceived risk knowledge.

Risk communication often relies on a fear appeal in order to motivate behavior change. As flight anxiety already has the flying public in fear, the Extended Parallel Process Model (EPPM) provides a useful framework to utilize in order to construct a useful risk message (Witte & Allen, 2000). According to the EPPM, a fear appeal or anxiety-producing message (or situation) will be processed either in danger, fear control, or with no reaction. This processing depends on the perceived severity and susceptibility of the threat as well as on the perceived efficacy provided in the risk message. This means that if no threat is perceived (e.g., no flight anxiety exists), there should be no reaction or change. If, however, both the perceived threat (in this case, flight anxiety) and efficacy are high, the outcome should be danger control, which is bon-adaptive (i.e., a reduction in flight anxiety). In contrast, if the fear is higher than the perceived efficacy message, flight anxiety will not be managed or will not change. The goal then, in message creation, is to provide a strong efficacy message that will lead to fear control, rather than danger control, and thereby ultimately to the desired reduction in anxiety and increased healthy behavior.

Using this theoretical rationale, a risk message was created that included a risk comparison and a strong efficacy component. The risk comparison (showcasing that less deaths occur from flying than from other forms of transportation) should reduce the perceived severity and susceptibility, and the efficacy message (that there is a means to look up the maintenance information about the airplane) should reduce the flight anxiety.

This study utilized a three-condition experimental design. The control condition featured a message about airlines' commitment to achieving passenger satisfaction and was meant to serve as a baseline of flight anxiety in a message that had nothing to do with safety. The message read as follows:

> Airlines dedicate themselves to serve their customers to the highest quality and satisfaction while also maintaining the optimal level of safety. In the air and on the ground, we're committed to bettering the lives of our customers, crewmembers and communities—inspiring others to do the same.
>
> We set out in 2000 to bring humanity back to the skies, when we noticed a lack of compassion, a missing human touch, in the air travel experience. It's what we're still doing today; only we've taken our promise below our wings and beyond our airports, bringing the customer service in the sky to charitable services on the ground. At our airline, we're not just committed to air travel. We recognize our responsibility to the world—to better the lives of our customers, our crewmembers, and the communities we serve, and to inspire others to do the same. This commitment to inspiring humanity is how we do business every day.

The flight anxiety with efficacy condition (Experimental Group 1) featured a two-part message about how individuals can check the maintenance of the aircraft they are scheduled for. The message is as follows:

> Aircraft safety is a high priority for all airlines. Aviation Maintenance Technicians (AMTs) assure comprehensive ongoing procedures that provide safety while in the air. The entire aircraft is examined and made sure that every bit and piece is up-to-date and maintained. Some of the duties during routine checks include: cleaning components, lubricating parts, inspection, checking hydraulics, etc. To ensure highest safety ratings, the entire aircraft is examined regularly and our well-trained technicians check that technology is up-to-date. This diligence ensures that flight remains the safest way to travel, even safer than driving in a car or taking public transportation. Now, it's easier than ever to check the maintenance on aircraft you may be scheduled to fly on. Simply

> obtain the tail number of the aircraft you are scheduled to fly on at the following website: www.faa.gov/aircraftmaintenance.com.

The flight anxiety without efficacy condition (Experimental Group 2) featured the same maintenance message as Experimental Group 1; however, it did not feature the portion of the message regarding checking the maintenance record of the aircraft. The message is as follows:

> Aircraft safety is a high priority for all airlines. However, with costs rising, sometimes airlines cut costs. Airlines often do this by cutting back on maintenance work for aircraft. By doing this, aircraft can continue making money instead of being out of commission for maintenance. When this happens, planes crash. Maintenance crashes are amongst the most gruesome out there and are fairly prevalent amongst all plane crashes. Most often, passengers do not survive these crashes. When scheduled for a flight, passengers are unaware of when a plane has been maintained. Therefore, every time you board a flight, you are playing Russian roulette with your life.

This experiment was initially tested in a laboratory with students that were frequent flyers. Although, these students were told to imagine this was a message from airport management that they were receiving while they wait for a flight.

Results show significant differences in flight anxiety between all three message types. For most, death thought accessibility (i.e., death salience) was highest among the efficacy message, followed by the message without efficacy and then the control message. Interestingly, there was no change in perceived airport risk for any of the messages. These results suggest that maybe airport messaging may not have an effect on anxiety as once thought, at least in a controlled environment. While we might think that giving the public the ability to check maintenance records might reduce anxiety, it very well may do the opposite. While not knowing surely is terrifying, is it scarier to know that your plane has not undergone maintenance for a while, or worse, it is just coming back into service after a maintenance problem? Perhaps not. An overflow of unlimited information and efficacy may be simply too much for passengers. However, one caveat should be considered with this data. Our experiment utilized a student population. While our samples *are* frequent flyers, these students are not flying passengers in an airport as those in the LAS study were. Therefore, some care should be given when interpreting these results as generalizable. Instead, perhaps this data can serve as a guide for future research in this area.

We as researchers need to give more effort to discovering how to decrease air rage incidents and whether this is an airport or airline issue. Because the fact is, air rage incidents *are* increasing. A quick anecdote search of incidents online shows a marked increase in the prevalence of air rage situations on places since the 1990s. And, while airports are doing everything in their power to help ease passengers with the design and management, it may simply be the nature of the airlines packing people in seats with virtually no personal space that may be the real culprit of air rage. Until airlines put passengers first instead of profit, the fear is that air rage incidents will continue to increase.

Chapter 4

Terror Management Theory and Plane Crash Survivors

I am not afraid of death, I just don't want to be there when it happens.

—Woody Allen

Surviving a plane crash is an experience that only a few have. This exclusive club includes people that are exceptions to the rule. Because, while surviving a plane crash is very possible, not many do. Survivors of plane crashes offer a unique look into what it is like to stare death in the face but live to tell about it. Through the firsthand accounts featured in this chapter, we see examples of heroism, changed lives, and community. But, we also see examples of behavior that are disturbing and hard to comprehend. All of these examples help to better understand how TMT and flight anxiety fit together. Even the most grotesque examples provide insight into how humans act when placed in a near-death experience.

IMPORTANCE OF CWV

One of the main ways to buffer death anxiety is through the management of a CWV. As mentioned earlier in chapter 2, the act of using a CWV as a buffer can be accomplished through socially acceptable and socially unacceptable ways. When a plane crashes, you do not have a lot of time to wonder about who on that plane is similar to you (i.e., part of your CWV). Therefore, you do not often see passengers turning against each other—they are too consumed with the management of their potential impending death. So naturally, passengers who find themselves in this unfortunate situation will choose the least cognitively taxing (read: easy) way in managing death anxiety—either through religion or management of close relationships. These two themes were quite prevalent in the accounts of plane crash survivors.

The two most common ways we see people handling death in their immediate future through accounts of plane crash survivors is through the adherence to some kind of religious belief and/or an immediate focus on the attachments they will leave behind. The easiest way is to start praying. Prayer was extremely common among passengers, interestingly, even among the "prior-to-this-moment" nonreligious.

On United Flight 232, multiple passengers stated that they were in the aircraft emergency situation for a reason. Flight attendants on this flight held hands and prayed—an action that several passengers partook in as well, with many passengers citing they felt God's presence. Brad Griffin even resorted to meditation. Passengers were very aware of how fast the plane was going, but after prayer and meditation, they all claimed to have no fear. Flight attendant Susan White describes in Lawrence Gonzales's *Flight 232* what it was like as she was saying the final words before crashing:

> "And as I'm yelling it," White recalled, "I'm saying the Lord's prayer in my head and focusing on the bright light, the tunnel—that swirling tunnel that takes you to heaven—the harps and everything peaceful that I had imagined heaven to be like." She looked out the window and saw that they were passing through a layer of clouds, so fluffy, so white, so beautiful, and she felt her love of flying once more. "Right before impact, I said, 'Okay, I'm in your hands, Lord.' And I had no fear at all. No fear. I took a deep breath . . ." And then she felt the devastating concussion and saw through the porthole in her exit door that a ball of fire had engulfed the plane. "And I calmly said to myself, 'I'm burning to death. That's how I'm dying.' And the fire was there. And then we started tumbling, and three times I remember it hitting on my door." (2014, p. 103)

Praying was also important for passengers on the U.S. Airways Hudson River crash. Passengers not only prayed for themselves; there were several accounts of passengers also praying for the pilots and others on the plane. Roberto Canessa, a survivor of the Andes Mountains crash, cited intense praying to God to not die. While praying gave most passengers comfort, on the Hudson River plane, a Buddhist on board claimed to have felt isolated and alone since he was not part of the majority of passengers that were part of the Christian faith. Even after the plane had crashed, United 232 flight attendant White stated she felt like she was put there by God himself to help passengers. On the other hand, United 232 passenger Martha Conent, a nonreligious individual, found herself bargaining with God to get her out of this situation. The Christian faith was also used by Roberto Canessa to make the difficult decision to consume fellow passengers that had passed away (citing Mathew 26:26 as his strength).

Samuel Aigbe, a passenger on the Kenya Airways flight, kept wondering if this crash happened because he did not do his usual pre-flight religious rituals. Once in the water, Aigbe heard fellow passengers calling on God for help and confessing sins, even as some were in the process of dying. Aigbe felt guilty for not living like God wanted him to and felt incredibly grateful for the second chance. Along with this newfound appreciation of life, Aigbe also had a strong desire to evangelize about his Christian faith.

So often attachments were built by other passengers through building relationships with other passengers, some of this was religious, but often it was not religious based. For instance, some passengers on United 232 were making plans to grab drinks when the crash was over. The act of making plans helps passengers to deny death by forming friendships and making plans after the pending horrific event provides some structure and awareness that this situation is only temporary. On the unfortunate Southwest Airlines flight, where a woman was partially ejected out of the window, survivor accounts state that the entire plane banded together to try to save her. And, on the Hudson River plane, a man had to swim to the other side of the plane, and upon arriving, a passenger gave him his clothes since the man that swam was wet and cold.

Many passengers also spent their time contemplating what life would be like for their families and friends after their passing, as well as a great deal of reflection. Carolyn Cross on United 232 had extreme clarity about what she wanted to say to her kids in a goodbye text once realizing the plane would be crashing. Like other passengers on United 232, she was also very concerned with who would take care of the kids and how their spouses would deal with such a tragedy. Cross's husband had a hard time coming to terms with the crash, which is not terribly uncommon, and now has a new appreciation for the fragility of life and does not sweat the small stuff, much like Cross herself. When Roberto Canessa was stranded in the Andes Mountains, continuing thoughts of his mother is what gave him the drive to survive. Sadly, his thoughts also turned to what life would be like for his then girlfriend, now wife, if he died. While thoughts of interpersonal attachments are very common in a crash scenario, sometimes the survivors found more interesting ways to deal with their situation and build attachments.

I suspect if you imagined yourself in a situation where your airplane was going to crash, your first thought would be to contact loved ones with goodbye messages and digital expressions of love. However, not all survivors handled the situation in this way. As a form of death denial, Kari Milford on United 232 did call her boyfriend; however, she did not tell him goodbye or the dire situation she was in. She simply told him she would be late. While this may have been a protection mechanism for her boyfriend, it also was a protection mechanism for herself. She is not accepting she will die, only that she would be a little late to her destination. Some passengers, during their self-reflection, chose to think negatively about their influence on their attachments. For instance, on United 232, John Hatch thought about his family as the plane was preparing to crash and focused on his regrets of not being a good father and husband. On that same flight, Martha Conent had similar thoughts about how she was a bad mother and wife. While this is definitely a sad way to spend your potential last moments on Earth, it is also a form of death denial. By pondering how bad of a person you were in life, this will ultimately help you feel better about death as well as how your attachments will handle your death. By imagining your attachments are better off without you, you are allowed to handle death with much greater ease. In fact, this thought process is often seen in individuals who experience chronic suicidal ideation as reasons to follow through with their intent (e.g., Harvell-Bowman et al., 2020; Joiner, 2007; Van Orden et al., 2010). Ultimately, feeling your attachments are better off without you is one of the ways these individuals manage their death anxiety in the moment of facing death straight on (Harvell-Bowman et al., 2020).

A more interesting survivor perspective comes from finding attachment relationships in nonhuman forms. Annette on United 232 found herself covered in insects after the plane crashed in a field in Iowa. Normally, insects, especially of the stinging variety, would give anybody a great fright; however, those insects provided Annette great comfort. She felt like these insects were her friends and she spoke to them as such. After the crash, Annette refused to be alone—she constantly needed human attachments. But, not all of these attachments are positive and built during the crash.

After the Kenya Airways crash, Samuel Aigbe had to find reasons to keep fighting. In his personal account of the crash and life after the crash, he cites responsibilities to his mother and younger brother as to what made him decide to keep fighting. In fact, his first thought upon being rescued was to ensure his family was immediately contacted because of a concern for his mother. However, Aigbe hoped that the passengers would have a lasting relationship, but that did not happen. As a form of potential death denial, the passengers did not band together postcrash; they wanted nothing to do with Aigbe or anybody else on that plane. If there were any kind of minor relationships, it would have been through the Nigerians, something that the Nigerian ambassador may have forced, according to Aigbe. While the survivors and families of the deceased seemed to support each other during the grieving process, after passengers were released from the hospital, everybody lost contact. The loss of contact with passengers is something that has bothered Aigbe greatly, and he mainly blames Kenyan Airlines for this. In fact, the entire purpose of his book can be seen as an attempt to reignite connection as stated by Aigbe: "I sincerely hope that others have recovered from the traumatic experience. . . . I honestly hold them all dear to my heart. . . . I strongly believe such a gathering would be of immense benefit to everyone. . . . This book is a cry out to the others to get in contact" (pg. 28–29).

The way in which passengers managed their immediate pending death is somewhat predictable given the TMT perspective. However, the nuance of differences within the survivors as well as how negative self-esteem was focused on by some suggests a more complicated view of terror management. Several felt they were not good to their attachments—regrets—very few said they were great people and it was okay to die. Passengers did what they could to manage death anxiety prior to the crash, but what happens when people are mere seconds from death?

When you are seconds from potential death, there are two types of people that emerge: people that accept it *or* people that deny it completely. We can see examples of both types in a variety of plane crashes. Many felt like they were not actually in the situation—the crash scenario they found themselves in was a movie or an event that they were watching—the event felt surreal. However, the surreal feeling did not last for long as passengers do eventually have to accept what is happening. Martha on United 232 was deeply saddened when she realized that that day was going to be the day she left this earth. In fact, once passengers realized what could potentially happen as they crashed, several put driver's licenses down their shirts so they would be able to be identified. This is the ultimate act of death acceptance. A United 232 flight attendant describes her experience:

> "Two-thirds of my body is in fire," she said. "I was engulfed in the flames. And I just said, 'Well, this is how I'm going to go," Death, it seems, can come to us tenderly. "It was the most serene moment of my life," she said. "There was no fear, there was no pain, nothing but total peace." And then Jan Brown was in limbo, suspended in her harness, neither awake nor asleep." (Gonzales, 2014, pg. 113)

As United 232 prepared to crash, passengers did the same. One passenger was even seen stretching, attempting to get his body to be as relaxed as possible before impact. But, not everybody was willing to accept crashing as easily. Surprisingly, one passenger told a fellow passenger he was not afraid and was thinking going down the emergency slide would be fun. The fellow passenger was terrified and spent his last moments before the crash contemplating how he would be killed, knowing this was surely the end. For the Andes Mountains crash passengers, there was no calmness at all: lots of questions about the experience of death still remained—some of the same questions that were found with passengers from United 232. However, as the Andes passengers looked down, they accepted the remoteness of the crash would almost certainly mean death, whether it be due to the crash or starvation. Passengers from other crashes focused on how they had had a good life and were quickly coming to terms with death. For passengers in the Hudson crash, many were not ready to accept death citing this was all just a bad dream and some United 232 passengers citing their spouses would not be able to care for their kids properly, so they simply could not die right now. Even Samuel Aigbe, who was cited earlier as wanting to survive for his family, reached a point where he was feeling extreme hopelessness and was in an intense fight between wanting to survive and doing the easier task, simply letting go. However, everybody has survived. And, now comes a very abrupt mental shift of survival and life post-crash.

I survived. Now what?

Once the plane has crashed, passengers now have to come to terms with the fact of what they had been mentally preparing for did not happen. Now, they must prepare for a new reality—surviving a plane crash where others may have died. Enter, survivor's guilt. The guilt experienced when surviving a traumatic event is a very real condition to anybody that has survived any kind of tragedy, and plane crashes are no different. The American Psychological Association defines survivor's guilt as stemming from not being able to prevent the event or not being able to save people that died (APA, 2020).

While survivor's guilt can happen after any traumatic event, it is more prone to happen with plane crashes for a few reasons. First, plane crashes are sudden and unexpected. Oftentimes these victims are at the most productive point in their lives, so they have not really spent a lot of time contemplating dying. Second, plane crashes are not orderly events. Plane crashes are messy and often feature scattered human remains and destruction beyond belief. In fact, people often find themselves quite stunned when visiting a crash site. Third, there is a lack of community. Typically, people are not crashing with a plane full of friends. Those who find themselves in a plane crash scenario are often among strangers, leading to no sense of community among passengers. Fourth, there is a strong irradiation effect, meaning that the crash affects communities from all different locations, not just the place where the crash occurred. Last, air crashes are mostly caused by human error, which can manifest among survivors as extreme anger toward the airline (Butcher & Hatcher, 1988). One way we can attempt to understand survivor's guilt is by looking at the psychological similarities it has with post-traumatic stress disorder (PTSD). Guilt-related trauma has been linked to increases in PTSD symptoms (Kubany et al., 1995; Lowinger & Solomon, 2004; Street, Gibson, & Holohan, 2005). Some of these linkages may even be different among the sexes. For instance, in sexual assault survivors, women experienced more guilt, whereas men experienced more anger (Galovski et al., 2013).

Control may play a role in these situations as passengers struggle to manage their terror. With surviving the crash and others' dying, the question of why and lack of control could be igniting death anxiety—making all of this much worse. The lack of control and lingering questions following a crash could be why some are obsessed with getting answers about the crash. The obsessive behavior of looking for answers may also be linked with their close relationships, as PTSD and survivor guilt can both put serious strains on these relationships. For instance, some crash survivors feel burdened by being given a second chance. Samuel Aigbe is often haunted by the prayers to God of the dying during his crash. Willy Phillips Jr. is still trying to understand, nine years later, why he was spared at age thirteen. And on United 232, one passenger could not understand why he would be spared, and a nun would not.

While survivor's guilt is definitely a negative side effect to tragedy, there is definitely a positive side. Many plane crash survivors have made significant life changes after their crash. For instance, after United 232 crashed, one passenger stepped into the cornfield, emerging from the rubble, and she immediately thought, "I am going to change a lot of things in my life" (p. 180). This sentiment was felt by many United 232 passengers—they felt like they were born again. After the Canadian crash, Carolyn Cross felt she survived her crash in order to bring her superbug laser to hospitals and clinics around the world, which she felt would ultimately change the way hospitals fight infections. She was certain her superbug laser was why her life was spared. Cross also had a new appreciation for normal life. And, after the Hudson crash, Lori Lightner left her job at Belk and joined The Red Cross, started an adoption process, and downsized her life with her husband. Willy, in the Alaska crash, sums all of it up well when he stated, "Every day when I wake up I think this is so infinitely better to waking up on the side of the mountain, so today is probably going to be a pretty good day."

Not all plane crash survivors use their post-crash life for good. In fact, for many, post-crash life can be filled with anxiety and anger. Oftentimes, we hear of heroic acts during plane crashes. People that saved others before themselves, and even giving the shirts off of their backs. But, that is not the full story of what *can* happen. Humanity has an ugly side, and unfortunately when faced with death, sometimes we turn to more selfish behaviors rather than healthier pro-social behaviors. For instance, when U.S. Airways Flight 1549 crash-landed in the Hudson River, there were heroic stories of passengers helping others. But, there were also stories of passengers stealing life vests and cushions from other passengers. Passengers activated their life vests prior to exiting the plane, making it very difficult to, in fact, exit the plane. And, while Roberto Canessa describes in his book that it was an act of devotion to have fellow passengers give their bodies up for nourishment upon death, the very act of eating another human being is quite grotesque.

After the crashes, some survivors discovered the uncomfortable nature of triggers that often ignites newfound anxiety, a residual side effect from the crash itself. Willy's plane crashed in Alaska, and he found that, months later, rain was a trigger. The rain was the last thing he remembered prior to crashing in the Alaskan wilderness. One United 232 passenger now describes a very strong startle reflex and consequently refuses to fly. This type of anxiety can often then turn to anger. And, this anger is often pointed toward investigators for not consulting the survivors during the investigation. Also, on United 232, Carolyn Cross found her anxiety turning to anger toward the media. She felt their stories should not have been focused on the crash, but rather the innocent bystanders that risked their lives to save hers. Samuel Aigbe's anger is pointed toward crash investigators, as he does not agree with much of the report and blames the corrupted African governments for compromising safety, which is why Aigbe believes the Kenyan Airways plane crashed.

THEORETICAL IMPLICATIONS

Survivors of plane crashes offer terror management researchers a unique look into what looking death in the face looks like, fully expecting to die, very quickly having to deal with that, and then living a life where you know what it is like to die. Typically, what plane crash survivors experience, in regard to flight anxiety, is less flight anxiety than frequent flyers who have never been in a crash. While this may be surprising, the idea of having *less* anxiety really makes quite a bit of sense from a terror management perspective.

Plane crashes are no doubt a scary thing. Why? Not a lot of people survive them. Additionally, the fact that while plane crashes are rare, dying in them is not, also makes you confront your mortality, something we all really hate to do. But, plane crash survivors have faced death. Death is no longer foreign to them and therefore a little less scary. And, if they survived a particularly gruesome crash, these survivors most likely feel like they can handle anything. For instance, in Carolyn Cross's crash in Canada, she stated, "I had always been fearful of crashing to my death. Now I'm actually not afraid of that anymore. It's rather odd. I had such a sense of peace up there." Samuel Aigbe refuses to let his crash taint his love of flying. However, keeping a peaceful mindset for Aigbe is a constant struggle for him. He has a bit of anxiety following turbulence and when flight anxiety really creeps back in for him is when the media reports about plane crashes, especially if the media reports a similar crash. Aigbe tries to gain a sense of control by taking on new precautions prior to flight as a direct result of his crash. The precautions help him feel less anxious. Others claim to have learned from the crash in a sort of post-traumatic growth. Oftentimes, we see passengers finding an increase in inner strength, discovering new possibilities in life, developing deeper relationships, strengthening their sense of spirituality, and even finding a greater appreciation for life—all examples of death anxiety-buffers from terror management research.

Death Denial

There are many examples of death denial in plane crash survivor accounts. One example is a failure to pay attention to safety messages, as cited by Martha Conant on United 232. While she cites she failed to pay attention to the flight safety message due to her status as a frequent flier, her lack of attention seems to be an act of denying death. This is something we have seen in research before (e.g., Lancaster, Bowman, & Harvell, 2015). Lancaster and colleagues showed that participants held high levels of fear, regardless of whether they were made aware they could survive a plane crash or not. This fear, coupled with the MS aspect of a flight safety message, proved too much for passengers. Recall was nearly nonexistent; they were not paying attention to the message. In fact, Lancaster, Bowman, and Harvell (2016) argue that fear *may* be a predecessor to MS.

Figure 4.1 views MS as more of an outcome when faced with a life-threatening event. This model suggests that if people feel like they can get out of the threatening situation, this helps immensely (Lancaster et al., 2016). And, this is where plane crash survivors are post-crash. They know they can escape and survive a plane crash, because they did.

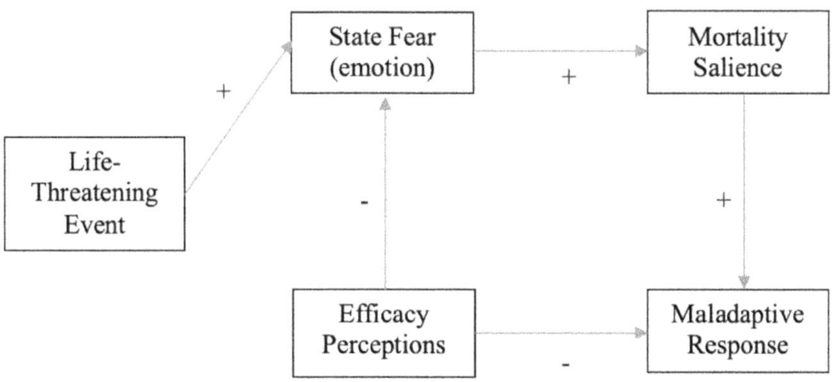

Figure 4.1 Proposed Conceptual Model for Fear, Efficacy, Mortality Salience, and Adaptive Responses. Note. As cited in Lancaster et al., 2016.

More overt death denials occur as well. When faced with death, Helen on United 232 said repeatedly that death is now nothing to fear. A group of United 232 passengers refused to believe the plane would crash until it literally hit the ground. They just kept telling each other that planes do not crash. As United 232 crashed, one of the flight attendants, Jan, just kept telling herself that she needed to be tough, calm, and not to give off any behaviors that might tip off the passengers to what might actually happen: "Then she squared her shoulders, forced herself into an attitude of professionalism, and began walking down the aisle, trying to figure out how to protect all those babies that people were holding in their laps" (Gonzales, 2014, p. 16). Ruth Anne, also on United 232, said, "and my fear was that we were going to have to go down that chute and that my skirt was going to fly up, and whoever was on the ground to catch me was going to see that I didn't have on pantyhose" (p. 37). Flight attendants on United 232 had to deny death in order to do their jobs and save lives. As they prepared to crash, they rehearsed steps to open the door, worried about how their family members would retrieve their cars from the airport parking lot, wondering which sisters would get their jewelry, and as the plane crashed, many focused their thoughts on getting to heaven and what it would be like.

Once the plane crashes, and you realize you are alive, it is difficult to deny all the death surrounding you, often in the form of dead bodies. But, as humans, even when you have death all around you, we all still find ways to deny it. When Annette crashed in the jungle, she made a point to focus on the beauty of the jungle that surrounded her and all of the *living* things—plants, animals, and even the bugs. Despite having all of these wonderful ways of thinking around death, there are still passengers like those in the Tenerife crash that simply refuse to discuss the crash. And, in some of their cases, they have avoided speaking about these details for forty years.

Symbolic Immortality

There are also accounts of plane crash survivors having a fair amount of symbolic immortality, that is, engaging in behaviors as an attempt to live on after death. The most infamous example of symbolic immortality is with the group that crashed in the Andes Mountains. Their story became famous as the individuals that ate fellow passengers to survive. While this act is hard for anyone to imagine, these men viewed it as a truly heroic act. The deceased lived on by providing nourishment to the living men until they could be rescued:

> It was an honor to say that if my heart stopped beating, my arms and legs and muscles could still be a part of our mission to get off that mountain, and that it

> could always be said that Roberto died trying to make that goal a reality. That was our greatest invention in the Andes: a generous death. (pg. 28)

Less grotesquely, United 232 passengers wrote notes that would be found after the crash. One such note reads as follows:

> July 19, 1989
> Aboard United Flight 232.
> Whoever finds this note,
> I have a new life insurance
> policy. The papers are in
> my guest bedroom closet.
> Jerry Schemmel
> (Gonzales, 2014, pg. 176)

While many planned for their attachments (and many called them), many others held back in fear that it would make their attachments simply too sad. The ultimate self-sacrifice, as those attachments are often the key to buffering death anxiety.

Chapter 5

Is the Media to Blame for an Anxious Flying Public?

Coauthored by John Panetti, Independent Scholar

Whoever controls the media, controls the mind.

—Jim Morrison

Every day, Americans sit on airplanes enjoying uninterrupted, sometimes relaxing, time to themselves. They may catch up on sleep, work (especially with the increase of Wi-Fi on aircraft), or just enjoy looking out the window at the land below. However, for some Americans, flying is not such a positive experience and can be a terrifying, and sometimes debilitating, task. As many as 25 percent of Americans suffer from a fear of flying (Airsafe.com, 2014). Living with aviophobia (fear of flying) can deeply impact how individuals function in their everyday life and can even impact their social relationships (Skolnick, Schare, Wyatt, & Tillman, 2012). Therefore, when individuals suffering from any level or form of aviophobia learn about plane crashes through the news, this has the potential to make their symptoms worse. However, not only individuals with a fear of flying have the potential to be affected. Decades of research have argued through several media effects models that news affects viewers (e.g., Cultivation Theory, Agenda Setting Theory, Framing, etc.). Given that viewing the news does capture attention from viewers and arguably has some effect on them, the possibility exists that certain types of news stories may affect some viewers more than others. Therefore, those viewers with aviophobia may find news stories about plane crashes to be particularly difficult. TMT offers some insight into what the psychological effects of viewing disturbing news may be.

TMT (Greenberg, Solomon, & Pyszczynski, 1997) states that one's deeply rooted concerns about mortality have an effect on his or her sense of self and social behavior. Every day individuals see graphic and disturbing images that can, if only for a second, remind them of their own social and physical mortality.

TMT, based on Ernest Becker's (1973) ideas about the denial of death, focuses on the psychological effects of pondering one's own death (Rosenblatt, Greenberg, Soloman, Pyszczynski, & Lyon, 1989). When this pondering occurs, it causes humans to feel terror, triggering them to take certain actions, behave in certain ways, or hold certain beliefs in order to overcome their own immortality (Rosenblatt et al., 1989). Chapter 2 provides a complete review and outline of TMT.

TMT research can help explain the flight anxiety that occurs after viewing plane crash news. When people are subject to images of airplane crashes in the media, they are confronted with subconscious feelings of their own deaths causing anxiety about flying themselves. This is especially true considering the catastrophic events of 9/11 inciting fearful responses from a great deal of people about flying. We can reasonably assume someone bombarded with the plane crash images that followed the disaster would have anxious feelings about flying because the overwhelming confirmation that flying is dangerous has been constantly suggested and validated through media presentation. Despite knowing that thousands of planes successfully ferry thousands of people every day without incident, the copious displays of disaster can create anxiety about our inevitable death potentially impending sooner than we had anticipated. Three different experiments give us insight into this troubling phenomenon.

EXPERIMENT 1

Experiment 1 examines the existential anxiety brought about by disaster coverage of plane crashes, something that research has not investigated to date. Research has consistently shown that news coverage has the potential to increase risk perceptions personally (Paek, Oh, & Hove, 2016) and in general disasters (Cheng, Hitomo, Otsuka, & Jeon, 2016); news coverage has even been shown to influence viewers to make health-promoting behavioral changes (Nabi & Prestin, 2016). As individuals are reminded of the death of others in a plane crash, they often contemplate their own mortality through imagining themselves in a plane crash. In turn, as TMT posits, certain cognitive changes occur when individuals are psychologically processing material after a reminder of death. When the salience of mortality is increased, there is an intensity of reliance on and defense of psychological structures that assist individuals in having meaning and significance in their life (Greenberg et al., 1990; Greenberg et al., 1997; Pyszczynski et al., 1996).

In order for these effects to occur, there must be some kind of priming of individuals regarding death, something that disaster news coverage instigates. Because individuals generally believe air travel is safe, when disturbing plane crash news occurs, their CWV (the safety of air travel) is threatened. Individuals with high self-esteem tend to respond less defensively to reminders of death (Greenberg et al., 1993; Greenberg et al., 1992; Harmon-Jones et al., 1997). However, those who have low self-esteem are less capable of coping with death reminders compared to those with high self-esteem (Simon et al., 1997). Therefore, the existing level of self-esteem serves as a buffer of existential anxiety when there is a decision whether or not one will continue to fly based on the information he or she gathers from news about air disasters. Because mortality salience (MS) is made prominent by news stories, those with low self-esteem will be affected by plane crash messages more (i.e., experiencing more anxiety) than those with high self-esteem. As individuals continue to read or view news regarding plane crashes, the level of self-esteem should affect the anxiety that one feels about flying in airplanes, such that those with high self-esteem will exhibit less flying anxiety than those with low self-esteem. Thus, it is predicted:

> H1: When exposed to plane crash news, death-aware participants with high self-esteem will exhibit less anxiety than death-aware participants with low self-esteem.

Because society often believes that news organizations are a credible source in reporting the facts about specific news events, these individuals are more likely to believe news about plane crashes when a source is revealed than when a source is not revealed (Bushman, 1998; Fukada, 1986; Nacoste & Hummels, 1994; Sherman & Lynn, 1990; Witte, 1994). Trust in public leaders and news sources are part of an individual's worldview. Taking self-esteem and worldview-based source credibility into account, each should play a role in the level of anxiety (high vs. low) one feels toward flying, such that as those with high self-esteem will have lower levels of anxiety when viewing a sourced plane crash story compared to those with high self-esteem viewing an unsourced plane crash story. Thus, it is predicted:

> H2: Death-aware participants with high self-esteem will report lower levels of anxiety related to flying after viewing/reading a sourced plane crash story relative to death-aware participants viewing/reading an un-sourced plane crash story.

Method

A total of 247 undergraduates (65 percent female, 35 percent male) were recruited from a large, Southern university. This split in sex is representative of the student population. Only participants who fly regularly (at least two to four times a year) were included to ensure relevance of the subject matter. A 2 (message prime: dramatic airline news/nondramatic airline news) x 2 (source: specified/not specified) x 2 (self-esteem: low, high) experimental design was used to examine the following dependent variables: fear of flying and death anxiety. Manipulation checks were performed to assess the strength of the MS condition.

Materials and Procedure

Experimental groups were run in a laboratory setting and participants were randomly assigned to experimental conditions. Prior to the message, participant's self-esteem was manipulated using bogus feedback from a PANNAS-X personality test (Harmon-Jones et al., 1997). Participants in the high self-esteem condition were given positive feedback while the low self-esteem condition was given negative feedback.

Participants assigned to the non-crash condition then viewed a nondramatic airline story that was either sourced (using a CBS News logo) or non-sourced. This story featured air travel becoming more expensive with fuel costs and the possibility of on-time arrival fees. Participants in the crash condition viewed a news story that was either sourced (again using CBS News) or non-sourced about the Continental Flight 4307 crash in Buffalo, New York.

Research has shown that MS effects are more pronounced when there is a slight delay (Greenberg et al., 1992), and a recent meta-analysis suggests a seven- to ten-minute delay (Burke, Martens, & Faucher, 2010). Therefore, the questionnaire began with a distracter task (e.g., solving a word puzzle) directly after participants were primed with death reminders. Participants then completed a series of death-related word stems that served as a manipulation check of MS (Greenberg et al., 1992), and then answered questions about flight anxiety and demographics.

Measures

Anxiety toward Flying

This measure was evaluated using the FASQ: Quantification of Fear in Various Flight Situations (Van Gerwen et al., 1999) assessing perceived risk associated with fear of flying as well as participant's views about their family or close friends flying. Skolnick and colleagues (2012) validated the FASQ questionnaire as having the ability to diagnose aviophobia clinically. Thirty-two questions inquired about levels of anxiety to issues directly and indirectly related to flying (1 = no anxiety to 5 = overwhelming anxiety). A factor analysis was used to determine combined flight anxiety measures; three different combined variables emerged. Turbulence flight anxiety ($\alpha = .967$)

consists of questions related to anxiety while in flight. Pre-flight anxiety (α = .936) consists of questions regarding an individual boarding or preparing to board an aircraft. Flight salience (α = .857) consists of questions related to a participant thinking about airplanes.

Death Thought Accessibility

Participants completed a series of death-related word stems that served as a measure of MS (Greenberg et al., 1992). The greater number of death-related words completed (six in total), the more death salient participants were. A t-test was used to measure death thoughts for the two conditions. There was a significant difference, t (245) = -2.360, $p < .05$. However, participants in the non-crash group (M = 2.09, SD = .996) completed more death-related word stems than the crash group (M = 1.79, SD = .973). These results suggest the presence of social death anxiety in addition to physical death anxiety and are discussed further below.

Results

The first hypothesis predicted that when exposed to plane crash news, participants with high self-esteem (M = 1.60, SD = .46) would exhibit less anxiety than participants with low self-esteem (M = 1.83, SD = .75). An Analysis of Variance (ANOVA) was used to test this hypothesis. Results show that a death prime and self-esteem are shown to only have an effect on flight salience anxiety (Turbulence Anxiety: F (1, 139) = 1.93, n.s., $\eta^2_{partial}$ = .014; Pre-Flight Anxiety: F (1, 139) = 2.71, n.s., $\eta^2_{partial}$ = .019; Flight Salience Anxiety: F (1, 139) = 5.11, $p < .05$, $\eta^2_{partial}$ = .035). Therefore, the first hypothesis is partially supported.

The second hypothesis predicted that participants with high self-esteem who viewed a sourced story about a plane crash (Turbulence Anxiety: M = 1.99, SD = .74; Pre-Flight Anxiety: M = 1.61, SD = .55) would hold lower anxiety levels toward flying than those viewing a non-sourced message (Turbulence Anxiety: M = 2.04, SD = .66; Pre-Flight Anxiety: M = 1.87, SD = .86). An ANOVA was used to test this hypothesis. Results show there was only significantly lower anxiety for turbulence and pre-flight anxiety (Turbulence Anxiety: F (1, 128) = 6.53, $p < .05$, $\eta^2_{partial}$ = .049; Pre-Flight Anxiety: F (1, 128) = 5.36, $p < .05$, $\eta^2_{partial}$ = .040; salience anxiety: F (1, 128) = 1.25, n.s., $\eta^2_{partial}$ = .010). Therefore, the second hypothesis was partially supported.

Discussion

Experiment 1 focused on the impact of media coverage of plane crashes having a number of societal implications. First, even though plane crashes are rare, disaster coverage can skew our perceptions of travel safety. This finding is important for the reputation management of airlines and for the global economy that depends on a trusted travel infrastructure. Second, and more importantly, watching disaster coverage may also influence how we interact with the world, even when the visceral images of carnage have faded away. Higher existential anxiety has been linked with greater intolerance of other cultures (Rosenblatt et al., 1989) and greater fears of societal alienation (Harvell, 2016). High levels of existential anxiety can subsequently impact, for example, how well we get along with people at work and how optimistic we feel about the economy.

There were a number of interesting findings. First, viewing disaster coverage instigated an increase in flight salience anxiety, especially for those who had lower self-esteem (H1). Other types of anxiety are also likely to happen when you are directly preparing to board a flight or when you are on a flight. This result supports previous TMT research showing the importance of self-esteem in buffering anxiety and also suggests that the mechanisms in TMT work with mediated messages. Moreover, death-aware participants with high self-esteem who view a sourced story about a plane crash held lower anxiety toward flying (H2). Therefore, results suggest that self-esteem and source do have an effect on anxiety, but only on turbulence and pre-flight anxiety. Those people with high self-esteem who view a sourced message about plane crashes have lower turbulence and pre-flight anxiety than those who viewed a non-sourced message.

The second hypothesis also contributes to a better understanding of source credibility and anxiety. Non-sourced messages contributed to higher anxiety levels compared to sourced messages suggesting source evaluation is important in TMT and is likely a component of our worldview evaluation. Future research should further explore trusted news sources as a function of fitting into a worldview.

Self-esteem and CWV also contributed to an unexpected, but highly interesting result—the presence of social death anxiety. However, not only disaster coverage increased MS, the condition using a story about increased airline prices also impacted anxiety. The manipulation check revealed that the airline price story produced a significantly higher anxiety level compared to the crash story. Manipulation check findings suggest that especially among younger people who may have money concerns, the threat of not affording a plane ticket created greater concern than the burning flames of the plane crash.

Physical death is the primary focus of TMT research, but social death is an unexplored yet highly useful segment of the research. While there is no set definition for social death, it can be defined as the loss of social status or the means by which people are judged to have worth in our society. CWV and self-esteem work as a function of status in society; status can be achieved by having things like a great job, driving a luxury car, living in a big house, or holding an important civic position. Social death is the loss of all status and things associated with that status, such as monetary accumulation. While physical death may be distant and abstract, social death is extremely salient to almost everyone. Social death appears to be quite prevalent among younger people whose social worth is not yet fully achieved and whose prospects may seem bleak.

Because these results suggest that the non-crash group was more death aware than the crash group, it is arguable that when there are competing types of death salience (e.g., socially death aware versus physically death aware), social death may prevail. In other words, social death awareness may be cognitively stronger compared to physical death awareness. This type of awareness has been shown inadvertently in other TMT studies (Fransen et al., 2011; Harvell et al., 2013; Martin & Kamins, 2010; Nisbett & Harvell, 2013; Wong, Nisbett, & Harvell, 2016). The differences between being socially death aware and physically death aware have yet to be explicitly examined by TMT research. Therefore, Experiments 2 and 3 examine this potential relationship further.

EXPERIMENT 2

Because Experiment 1 did not investigate the differences between text and video, Experiment 2 also takes into account the modality in which viewers receive their news. Experiment 2 tests whether seeing a plane crash on the news is more powerful than simply visualizing that plane crash when reading a news story about it. Research has shown differences between text and video for learning methods (Balslev, Degrave, Muijtjens, & Scherpbier, 2005; Lalley, 1998), but research on modality and plane crash news is lacking. Thus, it is asked:

> RQ1: How is flight anxiety different when comparing the text and video conditions?

Due to the emergence of social death in Experiment 1, Experiment 2 investigated this notion further using a new manipulation that has successfully shown the manipulation of social death (Wong et al., 2016). Additionally, because the anxiety felt would most likely be general flight anxiety, this experiment looks at overall flight anxiety rather than the segmented flight anxiety in Experiment 1. Thus, it is predicted:

> H1: There will be more flight anxiety present in death-aware participants when compared to non-death-aware participants.

Method

A total of 280 undergraduates (75.7 percent female, 22.5 percent male; Age: *M* = 18.96, *SD* = 10.36; Education: 92.3 percent Freshman, 2.2 percent Sophomore, 4.4 percent Junior, 1.7 percent Senior) were recruited from a large Southern university from introductory psychology and communication courses. The split in sex is representative of the university population. Like Experiment 1, only participants who fly regularly (at least two to four times a year) were included. A 3 (death salience: physical, social, control) x 2 (modality: in-person, online) x 2 (source: text, video) experimental design was used to examine flight anxiety. Manipulation checks were performed to assess the strength of the MS manipulation.

Procedure and Materials

Once consenting to participation, participants were randomly assigned to one of six conditions (Control Video: $n = 54$; Social Death Video: $n = 47$; Physical Death video: $n = 42$; Control Text: $n = 42$; Social Death Text: $n = 40$; Physical Death Text: $n = 51$). However, unlike Experiment 1, there were no significant differences between the death salient groups (F (5, 275) = 1.97, $p = .08$). Therefore, the death salient groups were collapsed into one experimental group ($n = 180$) and one control group ($n = 96$), which produced significant differences (t (193.13) = -2.54, $p < .05$). Participants in the control conditions either saw a video of news coverage about dogs flying on airplanes or a text transcript of the video. Participants in the social death conditions (pre-collapsed) either saw a video of news coverage about fuel costs increasing (the same video as Experiment 1) or a text transcript of the video. Participants in the physical death conditions (pre-collapsed) either saw a video of news coverage of a plane crash (the same video as Experiment 1) or a text transcript of the video. Participants were then guided to a set of questions regarding anxiety toward flying. Last, participants were guided toward demographic questions and then thanked for their participation.

Anxiety toward Flying

This measure was evaluated using the FASQ: Quantification of Fear in Various Flight Situations (Van Gerwen et al., 1999) assessing perceived risk associated with fear of flying as well as participants' views about their family or close friends flying. Thirty-two questions inquired about levels of anxiety to issues directly and indirectly related to flying (1 = no anxiety to 5 = overwhelming anxiety). Because this experiment measured overall flight anxiety, a factor analysis was not needed, as it was in Experiment 1. Reliability for this scale was excellent ($\alpha = .98$).

Death Thought Accessibility

Participants completed a series of death-related word stems that served as a measure of MS (Greenberg et al., 1992). The greater number of death-related words completed (six in total), the more death salient participants were.

Results

The research question asked how viewing a news story about plane crashes differs from reading a news story about plane crashes when looking at flight anxiety. An ANOVA test revealed there were significant differences between the text and video conditions (F (2, 275) = 3.17, $p < .05$). A Tukey post hoc test reveals there were only significant differences between the control videos. Because of this, the video and text conditions were collapsed for the rest of the analyses.

The hypothesis predicted there would be a difference in flight anxiety when comparing the death-aware and non-death-aware participants. An independent samples t-test examined the differences in flight anxiety levels between the control (n = 87) and experimental (n = 149) groups. There were no significant differences in flight anxiety between the groups (t (185.62) = -.94, p = .35). Therefore, H1 is not supported.

Discussion

There were no changes in flight anxiety from the text and video conditions, which is interesting since it is contradictory to Experiment 1, suggesting that it may not matter how an individual gets the news, the effects may be the same. Additionally, this effect may be unique to flight anxiety. The hypothesis examined these possible effects. Experiment 1 found there were some levels of flight anxiety present, but not all types existed. The second experiment sought to see if these findings would still exist when general flight anxiety is present and was not found to be the case. Regardless of text versus video, participants in this study just weren't scared to fly. While much of the concern seems to be over news media affecting viewers, it may be that it doesn't affect viewers as much as once thought. Experiment 3 investigates this notion further.

EXPERIMENT 3

Because Experiment 2 had differing results to Experiment 1, Experiment 3 served solely as a replication study to the second experiment. Therefore, the same hypothesis and research question was addressed.

Method

A total of 115 undergraduates (90.4 percent female, 8.7 percent male; Age: M = 18.84, SD = 1.07; Education: 62.6 percent Freshman, 27.8 percent Sophomore, 6.1 percent Junior, 2.6 percent Senior) were recruited from a large Southern university from introductory communication courses. Like Experiments 1 and 2, only participants who fly regularly (at least two to four times a year) were included. A 3 (death salience: physical, social, control) x 2 (source: text, video) experimental design was used to examine flight anxiety. Manipulation checks were performed to assess the strength of the MS manipulation.

Procedure and Materials

Similar to Experiment 2, once consenting to participation, participants were randomly assigned to one of six conditions (Control Video: n = 18; Social Death Video: n = 21; Physical Death Video: n = 16; Control Text: n = 21; Social Death Text: n = 21; Physical Death Text: n = 18). Like Experiment 2, there were no significant differences between the death salient groups (F (5, 118) = 1.65, p = .12). Therefore, the death salient groups were collapsed into one experimental group (n = 76) and one control group (n = 39), which produced significant differences (t (82.65) = -2.31, p < .05). Participants in Experiment 3 saw the same videos or text transcripts in the control and experimental conditions as participants in Experiments 1 and 2. Last, participants were guided toward demographic questions and then thanked for their participation.

Results

An independent samples t-test examined the differences in flight anxiety levels between the control (n = 34) and experimental (n = 68) groups. Similar to Experiment 2, there were no significant differences in flight anxiety between the groups (t (68.22) = .99, p = .32).

An ANOVA test revealed there were significant differences between the text and video conditions (F (2, 114) = 5.65, p < .01). Similar to Experiment 2, a Tukey post hoc test reveals there are only significant differences between the control videos. Overall, results of Experiment 3 replicate the findings of Experiment 2.

GENERAL DISCUSSION

Experiment 1 provided insight both theoretically and contextually. Theoretically, Experiment 1 produced a social death awareness finding that is just beginning to be understood. Contextually, Experiment 1 showed that plane crash news does produce certain types of flight anxiety. Experiments 2 and 3 investigated further the idea that social death may be a different type of death anxiety based on Experiment 1's results. It tested a new social death manipulation that has been used successfully in other studies (Wong et al., 2016). Furthermore, these experiments see if there is a difference between news that is gained visually and news that is gained textually. Experiments 2 and 3 violate Experiment 1's findings by showing that plane crash news does not affect flight anxiety as it did in Experiment 1.

Implications for Plane Crash News

The findings of these set of experiments indeed seem contradictory, however, the timing of Experiment 1 in comparison to Experiments 2 and 3 can shed some light on these results. Experiment 1 was conducted at a time when plane crashes were not occurring regularly. The study occurred before planes started regularly going missing (e.g., MH370), before planes were flown into mountains (e.g., Germanwings 9525), and before planes were being shot down (e.g., MH17). However, when Experiments 2 and 3 were conducted, MH370, MH17, and Germanwings 9525 all had occurred within the past couple of years. It appears that, while the plane crash news coverage may have been startling enough for Experiment 1 to evoke flight anxiety, the same video may not have been startling enough for individuals in Experiments 2 and 3, having potentially occurred because there was an increase in news coverage of plane crashes within the years leading up to Experiments 2 and 3, participants may have become desensitized to seeing graphic plane crash videos in the news. There may be a point in frequency where news viewers become numb to what they are seeing.

With the potential numbness in place, news organizations are then able to post more graphic detail in order to satisfy the attention spans of jaded news viewers. Future research should examine at what point viewers become numb to certain images. However, in the short term, the news does not appear to be causing rising elevations of flight anxiety.

While Experiment 1 examined sourced versus non-sourced messages, Experiments 2 and 3 did not examine this because the anxiety effects between sourced and non-sourced messages were not large. Additionally, messages received through the media are sourced, so the latter experiments wanted to focus on this. There were also no effects between text and video for Experiments 2 and 3. The idea that text is just as vivid as video suggests that how individuals get the news may not be as influential as once thought, arguing the vividness effects may be unique to coverage of plane crashes, but further research should be conducted to determine what relationship exists between the modality of the news and how it affects human behavior.

Last, since the emergence of online experimental tools, such as Qualtrics, there has been some concern among scholars that there may be differences among participants depending on whether they take it online or in the lab. When conducting experiments that need a lot of control, such as TMT experiments, there is a lack of knowledge regarding participant states. For instance, researchers have no idea if participants are getting interrupted during the experiment, if they are under the influence of any substance, and so on. With the increasing popularity of conducting experiments online, this study's results can offer support that in this sample the survey modalities did not produce different effects.

Theoretical Implications

Experiment 1 showed an emergence of social death when the control condition was more death salient than the experimental condition. Experiments 2 and 3 sought to replicate this finding using a new social death manipulation (Wong et al., 2016). While social death conditions did produce death salience among participants, social death conditions did not produce significant effects when compared to the physical death conditions. The inconsistency between the experiments is indicative of a variable that needs more study. When social death has been examined in TMT studies, research has continually shown this inconsistency (e.g., Fransen et al., 2011; Harvell et al., 2013; Martin & Kamins, 2010; Nisbett & Harvell, 2013). This study adds to the literature attempting to understand the social death phenomenon.

In all three experiments, plane crash news did a great job of evoking death salience. Even though in Experiments 2 and 3 the news coverage did not seem to evoke flight anxiety like Experiment 1 did, the effects of death salience can still wreak havoc on viewers' psychological defenses to this death awareness. In many ways, it could be a good thing that the over-salience of plane crash news does not lead to changes in flight anxiety. With those viewers that already have adverse effects to flying, only having to deal with death awareness and not a heightened sense of flight anxiety from news coverage *is* good news. One question that needs to be asked is, "What are the consequences for death awareness from plane crash news coverage?" The authors of this chapter suspect that the salience caused by plane crash news would be no more than the death salience caused by regular news coverage featuring stories on murders, shootings, and so on. Future research should look into the differences between the two before an analysis of the potential problem can be assessed.

Chapter 6

CNN and MH370

Journalism that Changed How Plane Incidents Are Reported

People often talk about parachute journalism, but one of the skills that you get when you are a correspondent is the ability to look at facts fast and work out what the story is.

—Richard Quest

The year was 2014. Barack Obama was president of the United States, ISIS became known as the new terrorist group to be concerned with, and in the spring, there was an Ebola outbreak making its way around the world. Flights were going on as planned, and the world commerce hummed on. In fact, on March 7, 2014, I was at LAS collecting data with passengers on flight anxiety. Little did I know the next day we would be introduced to one of the most notable aviation mysteries in history. Because, on March 8, 2014, Malaysian Airlines (MH) flight 370 would vanish while on a routine international flight from Kuala Lumpur International Airport to Beijing Capital International Airport. Approximately thirty-eight minutes after takeoff, the Boeing 777 aircraft lost contact with air traffic control, never to be heard from again. A jumbo jet with 227 passengers and 12 crew members had disappeared. At the time, and still today, we are all still baffled to think that a jumbo jet can simply vanish. News organizations were equally captivated by this story; on a quiet evening, aviation journalists were called in to immediately arrive at the studio for on-air analysis of the unfolding mystery.

On the evening of March 8, Anderson Cooper broke the news on CNN about the missing plane with the bare statistics—227 passengers and 12 crew members— first stating that air traffic control had lost contact with the airliner. According to Richard Quest, in his book *The Vanishing of Flight MH370*, he outlines how he heard the news. Richard Quest receives a message from the CNN Director of coverage informing him a plane has gone missing causing his blackberry to go crazy, as he had left the communication device at home to have a drink with friends celebrating his upcoming birthday. The messages were asking where he was, requesting he call the office immediately. Quest knew whatever was going on was something big. What wasn't coming through on his BlackBerry messages was coming through as even more urgent in his email. Quest quickly familiarized himself with the facts—MH370, the route, and the type of aircraft. Quest immediately knew that with several hundred souls on board, there had never been a fatal crash of a 777. Once finding out the basics, Quest contacted the CNN news desk in Atlanta informing them he was preparing to come back into work. Everybody knew it was going to be a long few days. CNN was quick and terse in their message back to Quest—get back to the office as soon as possible because they were going to need anything he could offer. On the way back to the studio, Quest researched the route and the weather in the aircraft's path. The plane went down in the cruise part of the flight, considered the safest part of the route. While the basic information was useful at first, speculations began shortly thereafter with the pilots. And, Quest was about to get the surprise of a lifetime. He had flown with one of the pilots—the first officer of MH370, Fariq Abdul Hamid. He found this out when a senior colleague forwarded a photo of Quest with the first officer in a Malaysian Airlines cockpit just a few weeks prior to the disappearance. This incident just got personal. But, the experience enabled Quest to provide *his* insight into what Hamid was like in the weeks prior to the disappearance, and no red flags were apparent.

Nonstop coverage of the missing plane went on for weeks. Months passed by before the search for the missing plane was not a top news story. Authorities searched for the plane for three years, with a second search in 2018. All turned up empty-handed. But, in 2015, debris started to wash up on beaches in the Western Indian Ocean. The first piece was found in Saint-André, Réunion, a flaperon confirmed to be from MH370. This debris was found west of the initial search area. More pieces of debris believed to be from the missing plane were found later in 2015. In July 2018, the Malaysian Ministry of Transport released their final report, which was inconclusive as to the cause or the location of the plane. While pieces of the plane have been found, we still do not have answers, and with the continued mystery comes conspiracy theories.

THE CONSPIRACY THEORIES

There are several theories out there that suggest different situations, some more believable than others. In 2015, *Wired* laid out what they felt were the most logical of these theories. The first of these theories comes from pilot Chris Goodfellow suggesting a fire in the cockpit. A fire, particularly an electrical fire, would have caused a loss of communication, a turn west toward Pulau Langkawi, and potentially the pilots to lose consciousness (Golson, 2015). The next theory from *New York* magazine argues that perhaps Russian Special Ops took the plane. In order for this theory to prove true, the electronics bay would need to have been accessed (located in the first-class cabin), during which an individual could have taken the electronics apart and sent some nefarious satellite data, somewhat plausible (Golson, 2015). At that point, the plane could have gone north into Kazakhstan and the 777 is currently being hidden (Golson, 2015). An email received by *Wired* suggests that perhaps someone filed a fake flight plan from an uncontrolled airport, pretending to be a small business jet—however, this theory does not answer how a Boeing 777 (and its passengers and crew) are hidden. Another theory suggests that perhaps this flight suffered a similar fate to MH17 and was shot down, but by the United States. This theory suggests that the plane may have been on a kamikaze mission and was secretly shot down before reaching its target (Golson, 2015). But, in order for this to have occurred, satellite data would have had to have been faked as well as a thorough cleanup of debris and keeping the passengers secret—something that is a bit unlikely, given the amount of people it would have taken to complete this *and* keep quiet (Golson, 2015). The plane could also be in Pakistan. Rupert Murdoch argues that the 777 was part of a jihadist plot against China (wired.com, 2015). Awaiting its next destination, Murdoch argues that the plane could be outfitted with a nuclear weapon for future use. We would be remiss to discuss conspiracy theories without mentioning those that find their way on Reddit. One such theory argues that the plane's demise could be due to supernatural forces—perhaps being taken by aliens, or a wormhole took it back to 1948 (Golson, 2015). Conspiracy theories naturally run abound directly following the disappearance. But, despite finding debris from the plane, there are still theories out there about the plane.

Recently, Ean Higgins (2019) wrote in his book, *The Hunt for MH370*, that perhaps Captain Zaharie Ahmad Shah parachuted out of the plane just in time to rendezvous with his lover that was waiting for him on a boat—a task that apparently seemed easier than getting divorced in the Muslim faith. The theory goes on to argue that fake IDs and a depressurized aircraft to kill the passengers, all led to a jump at 3,000 feet before the plane crashed into the ocean. Pretty far-fetched, but anything is possible, I suppose. Another, and somewhat more believable, theory suggests there was a sudden accidental cabin depressurization. If this would have occurred, Captain Shah could have been on break during the time of depressurization, leaving copilot Fariq Abdul Hamid alone with the controls—leaving him as the only one alive as he flew the plane to its eventual crash. Hamid's lack of oxygen would have led him to make bizarre decisions, explaining the rather erratic route, and finally ditching in the Indian Ocean (Rivers, 2019).

With the current technology, a cyber remote hijacking is not completely out of the question. Since 9/11, new technology was installed in aircraft allowing planes to be controlled remotely in the event of a hijacking (Davies, 2018). MH370 had this technology. Additionally, the cargo manifest did not make sense, suggesting there was something on board that someone did not want in China (Davies, 2018). There are still beliefs that the plane's fuselage had problems, something that is not new to the Boeing 777. In fact, six months prior to MH370 disappearing, airlines were warned by U.S. aviation watchdogs of potential cracks in this type of aircraft that could lead to a mid-air breakup or catastrophic depressurization while in flight, something the FAA warned about after finding a fifteen-inch crack in one of its planes (*The Week*, 2020). Of course, this theory does not explain why the plane supposedly crashed in the South Indian Ocean, a place not on its flight path. Some believe the plane is deep in the Cambodian jungle, something Ian Wilson (*The Week*, 2020) claims to prove with his intended visit to the jungle. Some other, less thought out, theories are that North Korea has MH370, or this was a murder-suicide and the pilot wanted the greatest aviation mystery ever, as explained by former Australian prime minister Tony Abbott (*The Week*, 2020). Regardless of the theory, the mystery surrounding this missing aircraft is as relevant as ever five years later. In general, plane crashes tend to ignite intense media interest, but a missing plane? Absolute media chaos. The missing MH370 plane has been described as one of the top unsolved aviation mysteries in history (Pujol, 2014). Because of the mystery surrounding MH370, the coverage options for this disappearance were limitless.

MYSTERY BREEDS INTEREST

What makes MH370 so interesting is the mystery it is shrouded in. The Malaysian government was hardly providing any information in the beginning days following the disappearance. And, when they did, the information was often incomplete and filled with uncertainty. Something that we as a human race do not handle well. We immediately speculate the worst.

For this crash, journalists typically focused on two strategies: (1) they created/covered sub/minor events that occurred and presented as new happenings that would lead to further reporting and (2) they looked to the past and future for events extending the scope of the incident (Sonnevend, 2017). In the first category, journalists would commonly use minor events to lead to further reporting such as when CNN received the cockpit recordings that led us to the moment that MH370 appeared to have turned off their communications.

In the second category, in 2018 the Malaysian government released a new report on the missing jetliner, introducing new coverage and new questions. This crash showed that journalists are overly eager to cover and create events, even when there are no fresh facts (Sonnevend, 2017). The Malaysian media had a wide range of types of coverage, but overall the media was starved of information, which made them more eager, which obviously led to more speculation. All of the journalists were baffled, so they constructed their own meaning which revealed the sociocultural positions of these media entities (Halim, 2014). A study examined three major newspapers in the United States, China, and Hong Kong reinforcing the idea that different media sources have different levels of power. High-power in-country media shapes the global agenda (Cui & Wu, 2017). All three of these countries had varying degrees of journalistic hysteria, leading other countries to follow. No information leads to speculation, and speculation leads to anger among the public. However, overall the media focused their stories heavily on placing responsibility and was the most important aspect of their stories, especially given that little to no information was often what they were drawing from (Bier, Park, & Palenchar, 2018). The unknown nature of this crisis made the media stories explode, and often with speculated content (Park, Bier, & Palenchar, 2016). However, MH370 was not the first plane to ever go missing. The media and public have always been fascinated with these types of events.

MISSING AIRCRAFT IN HISTORY

Americans have been captivated by missing aircraft for as long as one can remember. There have been countless missing aircraft and boats in the Bermuda Triangle that has captivated many by its mystery (and conspiracy theories). But, why are Americans more obsessed by this particular disappearance than other nations? I have to admit that I, myself, was equally captivated and was guilty of watching nonstop MH370 news coverage. Richard Quest, Mary Schiavo, and Les Abend were permanent fixtures in my living room.

Dr. Gail Saltz, a psychiatrist, explains that plane crashes can be terrifying not only because of the lack of control, but also viewing media coverage can help give us someone to blame for the tragedy, leaving us feeling more comfortable and relieved due to it no longer being a *random* event (Ford, 2014). Saltz argues that naturally flight anxiety will increase after viewing this type of media coverage, but the idea that people can just vanish may be even more terrifying than death (Ford, 2014). She continues to argue that being able to point the finger provides us with the need for closure that we all need. But, with MH370, nobody has received any closure, therefore leading to the continued intense interest in the story. And, with no answers, people begin to fear the worst. A plane crashing is rare, and one that vanishes is even more rare. Something like MH370 had never happened before on that scale, but Saltz argues that as you continue to watch media coverage about a rare event like MH370, it no longer feels rare. Some of the answer to our obsession may also lie in our nationalism, a component of our CWV. When we hear that an aircraft has gone missing, we are reminded of American sweetheart and Kansas native, Amelia Earhart—an aviator that went missing in 1937. Neither she nor her plane has ever been found.

Despite being a commercial aircraft, there are quite a few similarities to how we reacted to MH370 and Earhart's disappearance. One major similarity is both have a high number of conspiracy theories surrounding the incidents. People still hold out hope that both Earhart and the passengers of MH370 are still alive. For instance, there is a light that shines bright to the sky in Atchison, Kansas (Earhart's hometown), a light that locals believe will guide Amelia back home. On the other hand, many people all over the world still refuse to believe that MH370 crashed in the ocean. Both disappearances also featured lengthy and expensive government agency searches followed by searches conducted by private citizens. These disappearances also featured news headlines that contained immense amounts of speculation.

"Amelia Earhart Reported Missing in Pacific"

The Bristol Daily Courier

"Malaysia Flight Vanishes Amid Safety Concerns"

USA Today

"Technical Advisor to Amelia Earhart Believes Earhart & Noonan are safe after lost communication"

Honolulu-Star Bulletin

"Satellite Data Reveal Route of Missing Malaysia Airlines Plane"

Wall Street Journal

"Radio call raises hope that Amelia Earhart is alive and safe on land"

The Winnipeg Tribune

"Satellite Firm Says Its data could offer location of missing flight"

New York Times

"Amelia Earhart and Fred Noonan are pronounced dead when the search comes to an end"

Salt Lake Telegram

"Malaysia leaders face new fallout over plane search"

Wall Street Journal

While we did not have cable news or a twenty-four-hour news cycle in the 1930s, one could expect a similar frenzy of speculation to MH370.

Americans reacted to both disasters in similar ways: refusal to accept that it occurred, coming up with alternative reasons to the disappearance simply being an accident, and continuing to search, something we consistently see with Bermuda Triangle disappearances. There are still people out there that would like to continue the search for either disaster. And, thanks to today's technology, many still can via technological advances such as Google Earth. These are all classic examples of death denial. Both our and the media's obsession with finding the answers to these mysteries is very much a way to confront our own mortality. And, this type of coverage can be positive, with some viewers getting an adrenaline rush from the thrill from watching as argued by Saltz (Ford, 2014).

CONFUSION WITH MH370 MEDIA COVERAGE

While CNN certainly received a lot of attention for covering this story in depth, CNN certainly was not the only organization that reported on the missing aircraft. In fact, all of these organizations did at the beginning, just in very different ways and with very different information. Within the initial days following the disappearance, viewers were whiplashed with information. The day after the disappearance, on March 8, MSNBC reported oil slicks being spotted bringing hope to viewers that maybe the wreckage had been found. Unfortunately, two days later on March 10, CNN reported the slicks not being from the missing jetliner. With that disappointment came different news from Fox reporting that two men had boarded the aircraft with stolen passports, suggesting the incident may have terroristic ties. But, that evening, CNN reported that authorities believed it was not terrorist-related. Everybody was back to square one trying to figure out what happened but did not have to wait long. On March 11, CNN reported that the plane was off course when it lost contact with air traffic control. Then, the next day, CBS reported satellite images that were released from China suggesting shapes that looked like a plane. But, three days later, ABC reported that nothing was found in that area further stating that the images were released by China by mistake. All of these stories had a different frame, or perspective, depending on the network. Switching between networks, as I tend to do often, I was met with a barrage of conflicting information. This uncertainty, while completely normal for plane crashes, can cause unrest and anxiety among viewers. From a media standpoint, this constant stream of differing information always gave reporters and correspondents something to mull over and kept ratings high, especially for CNN, my personal favorite for all things plane crash.

CNN'S JOURNALISTIC MODEL FOR MH370

MH Flight 370 went missing around the time CNN's new CEO, Jeff Zucker, came on board at CNN. Zucker believed that CNN should do less stories, but cover the chosen stories extensively (Quest, 2016). CNN took this new motto to heart. MH370 was the *only* thing the network covered for weeks, with the exception of slight mentions of other news events. MH370 was front and center on every show on the network. CNN hired analysts to speak on air, hour-by-hour, about what they thought happened to the plane in whatever their area of expertise was (Quest, 2016). CNN aviation correspondent Richard Quest, Former U.S. Department of Transportation inspector general Mary Schiavo, and Boeing 777 pilot Les Abend became regulars on CNN as they were constantly in the living rooms of Americans. While this plane did disappear abroad, there were Americans on board, and Boeing manufactured the 777; America had a vested interest in this disappearance. This provided the perfect reasoning of why networks needed to cover this mystery.

While CNN received a lot of attention from other networks for their coverage, Jeff Zucker's new motto of exhaustive coverage of a few stories was clear from the beginning. But, while 24/7 airplane disappearance coverage was definitely getting noticed, it was not necessarily all good. For instance, Malaysia started accusing CNN of false allegations and fabricating stories about MH370 (Quest, 2016). *The Daily Show*, Larry King, and Erik Wemple at *The Washington Post*, all joined in on the criticism of CNN's coverage. But, despite this criticism, CNN was winning. Ratings were soaring, and Zucker's model seemed to be working. Richard Quest, at the time CNN's aviation correspondent, stands by this coverage: "These moments were the antithesis of the era of prepackaged, formulaic news coverage. It was why 24-hour news had been invented. Here the viewer was being invited to see firsthand the process by which raw news is analyzed and brought in to perspective" (Quest, 2016). While we are certainly aware from earlier chapters in this book that news coverage of plane crashes does increase death anxiety, perhaps the analysis and experts may help quell some of these fears and work to make death anxiety less. While regular news coverage may make anxiety worse, the CNN model of covering aviation disasters with experts and live-time analysis may be the way of the future for a healthier flying public.

PSYCHOLOGICAL EFFECTS OF TRAUMATIC NEWS COVERAGE

Missing aircraft are not the only aircraft events that ignite our interest, plane crashes also have a similar effect on our need for information. As human beings, we have empathetic and voyeuristic impulses that drive our obsession with disasters (Wilson, 2012). When we view this type of media coverage, it fuels feelings of relief within us that this event did not happen to us while also feeding our neuroses about these types of events (Wilson, 2012). However, with MH370, the fact that a jumbo jet could go missing when we can track an iPhone almost anywhere is hard to believe (Mason, 2014). But, it is important to remember that anything shrouded in mystery can breed obsession (e.g., Area 51). These types of events can breed social media addictions as well. For instance, social media was used by 80 percent of Malaysians and 68 percent of Chinese to receive their updates regarding MH370 (Changsong, Yiming, & Ahmad, 2017). Social media allows constant flow of news about a specific topic, even more so than twenty-four-hour cable news. MH370 was the first major crash since Asiana Flight 214 that crashed just short of the runway in San Francisco on July 6, 2013, that killed 3 and injured 182.

Generally speaking, news can be quite traumatic. Research has shown that increases in media exposure of traumatic events can lead to symptoms of post-traumatic stress (Bodas et al., 2015; Sampath et al., 2018). And, when news coverage is negatively toned, research has shown that people tend to also experience greater distress (Wormwood et al., 2019). The youth are particularly at risk for developing PTSD as a result of exposure to media coverage of traumatic events (Houston, 2009). Specific to plane crashes, higher anxiety was shown for those who read about plane crashes through perceived risk of victimization, but interestingly no relationship was found if, after viewing the plane crash news, these same people would rather drive than fly (Mo Bahk, 2006).

But, simply seeing this type of coverage is only part of the story. The amount of exposure can also breed anxiety. For instance, women exposed to news stories about cervical cancer were more scared about getting that type of cancer (Lemal & Van den Bulk, 2011). The more exposure they received, the more frightened they became. And, while there is no current record quantifying how much media coverage MH370 received across networks, we know that it was a large amount, worldwide, and an obsession of many, including yours truly. The amount of news one consumes has a strong relationship to how that person sees the world, something that Cultivation Theory helps us understand better. Cultivation Theory tells us the more we expose ourselves to television, the more influence it has on our beliefs about the world (Gerbner et al., 1980). Typically, research in this area looks at overarching patterns of television content or the relationship between television viewing and perception of real-world crime (Hetsroni & Tukachinsky, 2006).

Cultivation Theory can offer some insight into why plane crash news could cause an increase in anxiety. When you have journalistic coverage, like how CNN covered MH370, it is not surprising that 24/7 news coverage may cause viewers to experience an increase in anxiety, especially when the plane cannot be found. So, if Cultivation Theory is plausible, the twenty-four-hour journalistic model that CNN relied on for MH370 is *not* healthy. Sure, CNN's model may increase ratings, but it is a questionable ethical practice given the psychological impacts of this type of coverage for the flying public. However, there are some dominant communication frames that networks do tend to use. For instance, Rybalko (2011) found that the aftermath, cause, and human interest were typically what were used to discuss plane crashes. Readers in the same study seemed to be most interested in the attribution of responsibility and the cause of the crash, two things that we simply do not know immediately following a crash.

There is also the potential for lingering effects of anxiety caused by traumatizing media coverage. For those who have been in a plane crash or incident, this type of coverage can bring about hyperarousal and/or reexperiencing PTSD from that situation (Collimore, McCabe, Carleton, & Asmundson, 2008). For instance, research supports that media coverage on terrorism increases anxiety (Slone, Shoshani, & Baumgarter-Katz, 2008). In fact, there is almost always increased viewing of traumatic events due to human nature and Dependency Theory (Ball-Rokeach & DeFleur, 1976). Dependency Theory states that we have a dependency on media during traumatic events because we need to (1) share collective emotions, (2) enhance control, and (3) receive information, something that with social media can be constant (Ball-Rokeach & DeFleur, 1976). We saw similar effects with the initial coverage of the Covid-19 Pandemic.

In early 2020, the world became a breeding ground for the latest pandemic, a new coronavirus named Covid-19. Once this virus began to take hold in America, the media was nonstop virus, something that felt eerily similar to MH370 coverage, and with just as much death salience, if not more. At the time of writing this book in 2020 during this pandemic, effects of this media coverage are still being investigated, but preliminary data suggests a grim picture for our psyches. It appears as though Western media coverage caused problems all over the world. For instance, this media coverage provided great anxiety among the Chinese in both China and abroad, leading to troubling racial discrimination among Asians throughout the world (Wen, 2020; Wen, Aston, Liu, & Ying, 2020). In Greece, depressive symptoms were highest with those individuals overexposed to media about Covid-19 (Skapinakis et al., 2020). And, the constant change in information led to mistrust in the media in Sweden (Irwin, 2020). But not all of this coverage was bad. In America, the constant urban-focused coverage caused rural communities to follow Covid-19 protection protocols more stringently, ultimately saving lives (Kim, Shepherd, & Clinton, 2020). While not all bad, this type of media coverage can be quite damaging to the psyche and overall well-being of our mental health.

Media owners and journalists are in quite a predicament. They need ratings. Ratings are what make the networks money. Stories like MH370 and other aviation disasters/mysteries provide that tenfold. And, when you have a mystery that has golden journalistic potential, as a business, you have to pounce. But, what is currently not part of this business model is any focus on the psychological health and well-being of the public that gives them these ratings. The current model must begin to take into account the psychological well-being of consumers. To not do this is ethically irresponsible.

Chapter 7

Fixing the Current Journalistic Model

Journalism can never be silent: that is its greatest virtue and its greatest fault. It must speak, and speak immediately, while the echoes of wonder, the claims of triumph and the signs of horror are still in the air.

—Henry Anatole Grunwald

On June 1, 1980, Americans were introduced to CNN. This was the first time that news consumers could access the news on television twenty-four hours a day. Prior to this, Americans were relying on thirty-minute broadcasts on the three major networks: ABC, NBC, and CBS. While at first, this was a hard sell for Americans, CNN really started to gain attention during their live coverage of the Persian Gulf War in 1991 (History.com, 2009). It was at this point that Americans really started to recognize the importance of cable news. A thirty-minute broadcast was not able to provide the in-depth live coverage that a twenty-four-hour news option like CNN could. Today, several options for twenty-four-hour news exist, many with a political slant. In addition to CNN, there is Fox News and MSNBC. Additionally, there are also international sources such as the BBC and Al Jazeera English. All of these networks typically follow the same journalistic model, but as mentioned in the previous chapter, CNN has recently changed their model to focus more in-depth on specific stories rather than small snippets of a larger amount of stories.

Today cable news heavily relies on the panel format for their coverage. Panels typically feature people with different perspectives, something that is sure to bring lively opinions and often feature disagreements (Farhi, 2018). The panel format is also less expensive than journalism in the past as it is quite expensive to send reporters and crew to where the news is happening (Farhi, 2018). And, now viewers have come to expect their news to be served with a side of opinion, something that seems to hold the attention of viewers much more than newspapers. Opinion news is the new frontier. Today, half as many journalists work at newspapers as did a decade ago (Farhi, 2018). Another characteristic of today's cable news is that these journalists are often tied to reporting under a particular ideology (Perloff, 2014). So, the twenty-four-hour news networks focus on targeting viewership within a specific partisan framework (Hmielowski et al., 2015). But, plane crashes are not exactly partisan. Plane crashes open up the possibility for networks to showcase their stories to a much wider audience. As reflected in their ratings, everyone was watching CNN's coverage of the missing Malaysian plane, regardless of political affiliation, because CNN was the one network that covered this story more in-depth and with more analysis than any other cable news network. At the end of the day, the hosts of cable news shows are essential to the branding and marketing of the network (Landreville & Niles, 2019). The cable news networks of today switch back and forth between objective reporting and subjective commentary (Landreville & Niles, 2019). However, this is problematic because it can encourage outlet-favored misunderstandings, despite having knowledge of the evidence (Garrett et al., 2016). In politics, we see journalistic models trending toward the extreme and conflictual on cable news (Padgett et al., 2019).

The answer as to why this is the model journalists follow may be in how we teach journalism. For instance, today journalism students must develop skills to be able to assess what they read such as dissecting hoaxes, assessing credibility, social media sources, and ethical and journalistic transparency (Glisson, 2019). Being a journalist today is much more difficult with the technological advances when compared back to the early 1900s or even the 1950s. Today, the media has had to fight for credibility with attacks from President Trump and accusations of being "fake news." Furthermore, today's news consumers *want* analysis, not just the facts. Journalists are expected to report the facts on the ground and while explaining them, not to oversimplify—a daunting task given the wide range of cognitive ability among consumers (Klein, 2019).

With the twenty-four-hour cable news cycle and the internet, journalists today have constant deadlines. They are often expected to be immediately tweeting or livestreaming the news, something that their journalistic ancestors never were faced with (Klein, 2019). The journalists of yesterday had time to digest the news and get facts and sources straight prior to sharing it with the world. There is no time for that today in the competing market of networks—you must report immediately so that your network owns the story. There is rarely time to digest the information. With this kind of environment, journalists often make errors in their reporting and have to backtrack in later stories. This report-immediately model is simply not sustainable for the integrity of journalists. When journalists make mistakes the public becomes uncertain, and with uncertainty comes anxiety. There must be a change in the current model.

Changing the current journalistic model is not anything new. As society has changed, so has journalism. But, even journalists are starting to take note of the problem and calling for a change in the cable news model. Judy Woodruff, Special Correspondent for MacNeil/Lehrer Productions, demands a new business model that would bring in higher revenue that would enable networks to pay for high-quality journalism. Similarly, George Niesen, Vice President and Managing Editor for Kagan Research, wants journalists and networks to focus on getting the whole story quickly, but much more in depth. And, David Payne, Senior Vice President for CNN News Services and General Manager for CNN.com, suggests that online versions of cable news should be used as a complimentary source—a way to reach even more viewers—not a completely separate entity.

This model of journalism has the potential to make any anxiety induced by traumatic news stories much worse. Watching anything for twenty-four hours can be problematic for the psyche. While the panel format definitely provides viewers with a wide range of perspectives, disagreements on these panels can often end in shouting matches, something that can be seen on all of the major cable networks. The confusion that viewers may have also can play a role in this anxiety. A recent contributor to cable news anxiety is President Trump's constant attacks on not only the media networks but also individual reporters, causing doubt among viewers. In today's media environment, people do not know who to believe, something that was evidenced in the press briefings during the Coronavirus pandemic (Terkel, 2020). If you cannot trust the media for information, who do you trust? The kind of uncertainty manifested by distrust has the potential to throw any news consumer into a paranoid existential crisis. And, in a world already ripe with mental health concerns, this is certainly troubling. But, there is something journalists can do to help.

A NEW MODEL OF JOURNALISM

The key to finding a new way to think about cable news journalism is really twofold: (1) networks need to produce enough ratings to generate high revenue, but (2) they also need to be ethical in what they are reporting. And, these ethics aren't your grandmother's journalism ethics. Today, source credibility is more important than ever. And, while we need to report the facts, we need to do so in a way that always has the consumer's psychological health in mind. With the ever-present death salience with not only aviation disaster news, but all news, here are some recommendations on what journalists can do to report the news in a better way, from a psychological standpoint, when reporting on plane crashes and other traumatic events (table 7.1).

The first step to a better journalistic model is to eliminate the speculation, knowing that in the beginning hours of a plane crash or traumatic event, doing this will be extremely difficult. However, the end game is worth it. When journalists focus on facts, and the analysis of those facts, viewers will feel less uncertainty. And, when there is a desire to speculate, draw parallels to past events. Drawing parallels will provide new content *and* provide viewers with the comfort that whatever is being reported on has occurred before. In fact, even with the mystery and shock surrounding MH370 going missing, it certainly was not the first aviation mystery. Viewers can take comfort in that.

Second, journalists need to treat breaking news as breaking news, but not weeks of nonstop 24/7 coverage of the same material. Once a few days have passed, and you get past the initial event, devote fifteen minutes an hour to the story, but report on other things in the world. This change in coverage will help viewers realize that, while this new event is scary and uncertain, the world is still turning. Other stories will also serve as a break for the psyche and further help to curb anxiety. The new journalistic approach could also help with ratings. Because viewers are not inundated with constant coverage, viewers will crave news about the new event, potentially causing them to tune in more frequently. Third, networks would benefit from employing psychologists and have them on air to discuss the impact these events have on the public. For instance, this occurred on CNN and other networks with the Coronavirus pandemic. While coverage was constant and quite grim at times, networks did a great job of having psychologists on air to discuss what the public could do to protect their psychological health. Networks need to continue this model for plane crash news. Last, networks really should rely on their online outlets for more complementary, in-depth analysis while referencing television content. CNN is currently doing this; however, other networks attempt, but the attempt is rather haphazard. Relying on online modalities enables these networks to reach a wider swath of the population. And, putting more emphasis on the network website could potentially bring more people to the network, further boosting ratings. But, journalists are not the only ones to blame. We need help from the aviation professionals as well.

Table 7.1 Steps to a Better Journalistic Approach

1. Eliminate any speculation.
2. Treat breaking news as breaking news, but not nonstop 24/7 coverage weeks later.
3. Have psychologists on air to talk about the impact of these events.
4. Rely on online sources for more complementary in-depth analysis.

HOW AVIATION PROFESSIONALS HANDLE CRASHES

In the initial hours of a crash, the airline, involved airports, and the NTSB are scrambling to manage the crisis that has just been thrust upon them. While the NTSB is getting a team ready and on site to investigate, the airlines and airports often have to work together to manage the public crisis. The good news is most major airlines that have had disasters in the past have plans in place. These plans typically include the following: (1) family assistance centers, (2) a telephone hotline for families, (3) the designation of specific employees for individual families, (4) on-site grief counseling, and (5) a JIC (joint information center) for airline personnel and investigators with a nearby media room for reporters (Mintz, 2014).

After 9/11, both United and American airlines relied heavily on their websites to manage that crisis involving several of their aircraft. They provided immediate facts, provided condolence messages, and links to relief organizations (Greer & Moreland, 2003). The airlines handled the situation right and everybody blamed the terrorists, not the airlines. Company websites provided airlines a chance for an immediate response as well as a way to provide frequent updates. They were not reliant on the media to get their message out—they controlled the message, something that is incredibly important during a crisis such as an aviation disaster. Following a crash, airlines often already have an uphill battle convincing passengers their planes are safe (Bryant, 1994). And, while we like to think our airlines in America have these crisis plans in place, Malaysia Airlines showed us how bad a public relations disaster could truly be following a crash.

A HARD LESSON IN PUBLIC RELATIONS

The year 2014 was a rough one for Malaysian Airlines. In March 2014, they lost a Boeing 777 plane headed for Beijing that is still missing at the time of writing this book. A few short months later in July, another one of their Boeing 777 planes had an incident. MH17 was shot down while flying over Eastern Ukraine. While MH17 had differences from MH370 (namely they knew where it was), the incident provided an opportunity for the airline to redeem themselves after their embarrassing response to the MH370 disaster.

When the situation became known that MH370 was not making its scheduled landing in Beijing and worse, nobody knew where the plane was located, the world quickly realized Malaysian Airlines was not prepared for this kind of crisis which became painfully apparent when the airline did not exactly respond to the crisis immediately, and when they did, they withheld information in a way that made the world highly suspicious of the government-owned airline (Roach, 2015). To make matters worse, Malaysian Airlines was seriously lacking in their sensitivity toward the families of MH370 passengers. For instance, after sixteen days of endless waiting, the families received the following text from the airline:

> Malaysia Airlines deeply regrets that we have to assume beyond any reasonable doubt that MH370 has been lost and that none of those on board survived. As you will hear in the next hour from Malaysia's Prime Minister, we must now accept all evidence suggests the plane went down in the Southern Indian Ocean.

A text message. Not exactly the *best* example of public relations during a crash. And, families, along with the rest of the world, were rightly offended. When airlines do not have solid crisis plans, as was clearly the case with Malaysian Airlines, the lack of information causes the media to report false information and also have no plan.

But, it is possible that Malaysian Airlines was just caught off guard. Going through the MH370 crisis enabled the airline to put together a comprehensive crisis plan so they would not be such a mess the next time a disaster occurred. Unfortunately, Malaysian Airlines would have this tested much sooner than anyone would expect. Just a few months after the disappearance of MH370, MH17 crashed. But, the chaotic scenes following the disappearance of MH370 were definitely a thing of the past. Is it possible that Malaysian Airlines learned from their mistakes? It appeared so. The airline seemed much calmer and full of confidence this go around (Watts, 2014). Following the MH17 crash, Malaysian Airlines held regular press conferences, and while this was not a missing plane, the airline did appear to have a better handle on communicating with the public about the disaster (Azmi et al., 2016), something we can all hope is a mainstay for the government-owned airline in the future.

COLGAN AIR 3407

The last American commercial airliner to crash holding passengers belonged to Colgan Air, owned by Pinnacle Airlines, a regional airline. Like most regional airlines, they typically operate in codeshares with larger airlines, meaning the regional airlines are operators of the aircraft owned by the larger airline. In the case of flight 3407, this Bombardier Dash-8 Q400 regional aircraft belonged to Continental Airlines. The plane crashed on a cold evening in Buffalo, New York in February 2009. That means, that at the time of writing this book, there has not been a fatal American commercial airline crash involving passengers in over a decade. Because the crash site featured a prominent Continental Airlines logo on the tail engulfed in flames, it was already fairly difficult for the media to get across to the public that

Continental Airlines was not responsible since they were not in operation of the aircraft (Minkel, 2009).

Even though regional airlines are not major airlines, how Colgan Air handled this disaster was nothing more than a wonderful example of public relations. In the week following the crash, the airline released a total of ten statements and an FAQ (Minkel, 2009). Interestingly, even though the airline was not immediately aware of the cause, they were completely upfront about that with families of the passengers, and consequently the media followed suit. Because of this honesty, safety procedures changed as a result of this crash making air travel much safer. Overall, airlines need to focus on purchasing "safe" planes, and while sustainability is important as is the case with the Boeing 787, it is vital that airlines also focus on the crashworthiness of the plane (Smith, 1999).

BOEING 737-MAX

Throughout history, there have definitely been times when certain aircraft models have been grounded—the DC-10, Concorde, Boeing 747, Airbus 380, and even the new Boeing 787 Dreamliner. Other than the DC-10 and the Concorde, all of these have been temporary. The aircraft manufacturers quickly corrected the problems and the planes were back in service. And, the Boeing 737-MAX just recently joined this group beginning service again in December 2020. Few aircraft groundings have caused the anxiety that grounding the 737-MAX did. Generally speaking, the 737 is the workhorse of the skies. This narrow-bodied, short-range aircraft was a common sight for domestic passengers. And, the 737 had an amazing safety record. Americans felt safe on the 737.

The 737-MAX is a fourth generation 737, redesigned to be more fuel efficient and had its first flight in 2016. But, as airlines were quickly buying up the new aircraft, the 737-MAX began to have problems. The first problem arose in October 2018 with Lion Air Flight 610 that crashed after takeoff from Jakarta. After came a flurry of concerns from both the FAA and the Allied Pilots Association. After an investigation, the FAA concluded there was a fatal flaw in the MAX that would cause future crashes (Hemmerdinger, 2019).

Yet, the MAX continued to fly. Then, less than a year later, in March 2019, Ethiopian Airlines Flight 302 crashed after takeoff from Addis Ababa Airport. This crash was caused by the same fault that caused Lion Air Flight 610 to crash. Boeing officially had a big problem. Three days later, the FAA *finally* grounded the MAX. Cue the media storm. Boeing was in one of their largest public relations failures. Boeing was *severely* delayed in its apologies and often conveyed confusing messages. They apologized for the safety while vowing to update the plane. But, at the end of the day, Boeing was simply unable to convince people they cared and that caused quite a bit of anxiety for passengers (Baker, 2019).

Boeing was not about to give up. After the board of directors saw how poorly Boeing CEO Dennis Muilenburg handled the crashes (e.g., publicly blaming the pilots), he was excused from his position in December 2019 (Masunaga, 2019). Since then, Boeing has focused on making the required changes to see the MAX take to the skies once again. Recently, the FAA has taken steps forward on the road to recertifying the MAX (Schaper, 2020). Despite the changes, passengers are understandably anxious about hopping on board the MAX. Only time will tell if passengers will still feel comfortable on this aircraft, and with Boeing.

ANXIETY

Obviously, the way MH370 was handled led to an overall increase in anxiety all over the world. And, a lot of what was being communicated to the media was wrong, causing journalists to backtrack, contradict, and generally confuse viewers.

At the beginning, withholding information was necessary. In fact, the NTSB typically withholds all information until after their investigation is complete (a process that normally takes over a year). But when airlines lie about information and continue to change their story, the public will get anxious. Consequently, when airlines do not communicate, the lack of communication also breeds anxiety. The families of crash victims are extremely vulnerable immediately following a crash and need almost constant communication. When airlines engage in all of these activities, it makes the journalist's job next to impossible. So, now not only are the airline's public relations' mistakes, following a disaster, affecting the families of crash victims, but also are affecting the greater flying public, thanks to mass media.

The way Colgan Air handled the 3407 disaster is a great example of how to lower anxiety. Therefore, I recommend that aviation professionals follow three steps to help tame anxiety among the flying public following a crash (table 7.2).

Table 7.2 Steps for Aviation Professionals

1. Overcommunicate.
2. Daily Press Briefings.
3. Refer to Colgan Air 3407 as a public relations model.

The first step is to overcommunicate relevant details. This means daily communication with families of the crash victims and the media. Nobody has ever complained about *too* much communication during a disaster. The second step is to hold daily press briefings. Even if there are not any new findings in the crash investigation, having a space where you can communicate that while also having a time daily where the media can have their questions answered allows the airlines to control the message better. The third step is to rely on Colgan Air as a model for handling aviation disasters. Imagine how much better things could have been if Malaysian Airlines had followed this model.

There are specific things that journalists and aviation professionals can help do to decrease anxiety among the flying public. The one that bridges all entities in a disaster is communication and communicating accurately. By doing this, we feel like we are in the know, and this feeling naturally helps us feel less anxious. But, not all of this anxiety is wrapped up in the actions of journalists and aviation professionals. The scary part is that we could be involved in a crash any time we step foot on an airplane. And, when we board that plane, we give up complete control on whether we safely arrive at our destination *or* we crash into the earth at dizzying speeds. So that begs the question as to what the flying public can do to help curb some of this inevitable flight anxiety.

Chapter 8

What Can the Flying Public Do?

Flying itself may require no magic, but fearless flying relies on a collective delusion of occult proportions.

—Will Self

Let's be honest. Airline professionals have their hands full. Commercial air travel is not the prestigious, exclusive mode of transportation that it was in the 1950s. Flying became something of a necessity, especially for global businesses. As the increase in travel became more commoditized, airlines began to pack more passengers on the planes. On a domestic flight today, the free meals of the 1980s are a thing of the past. And, specialty airlines like Midwest Airlines, which featured warm chocolate chip cookies and an all-business class cabin, were bought up by budget airlines. In this case, Denver-based Frontier Airlines. And, chocolate chip cookies aren't *exactly* budget-friendly, so those are a distant memory, much to the dismay of frequent Midwest Airlines cookie lovers, including yours truly.

Today, air travel caters to the cheap passenger with options for "basic economy" on major airlines and dirt cheap fares (e.g., $25 one-way) on airlines like Spirit, home of the "base-fare." On these airlines, nothing is free. Want to pick your seat? Want a glass of water? It will cost you. Some of these low-cost airlines even charge to use their overhead bin space. Currently, they aren't placing passengers in that space, but only time will tell if that remains true. Passengers no longer wear their Sunday best to fly. When boarding a plane today, you are more likely to see people in workout attire or pajamas.

The crowding, lack of respect, and unhappy passengers about being nickel and dimed are already set up for anxiety in flight. Add alcohol to the mix, and you immediately start to wonder why anyone would want to work for an airline, let alone *in* an airplane. And, with all of these obstacles, it makes sense that the flying public are walking balls of anxiety. Something that was clear at research conducted at Las Vegas International Airport in 2013 (Harvell et al., 2016).

A LOSS OF CONTROL

When we board an airplane, we give up a certain amount of control. In the same line of thinking, we also do not have control over when we will die. As noted throughout this book, both produce very similar anxieties. When there is a loss of control, research has shown an increase in anxiety related, but not limited to, sports injuries (Kleinert, 2002); eating disorders (Byrne et al., 2020), internet addiction (Capetillo-Ventura & Juárez-Trevino, 2015), and parent's reactions to children with cancer (Boman, Lindahl, & Björk, 2003). In fact, women tend to be more phobic than men when it comes to flight anxiety (Ekeberg et al., 2014). Whenever there is a loss of control (or perception of that loss) in *any* situation, anxiety increases. So, getting on a plane should really be no different; a plane is a natural situation for anxiety to breed.

This loss of control seems to be acknowledged by the flying public. Will Self, frequent anxious flyer, notes, "The only flights on which I've ever felt at complete ease are the ones where I've been in the cockpit with the pilot" (Self, 2014, p.70). This makes sense. By being in the cockpit, you gain a sense of calmness because you are *watching* the plane being flown. You can see it. You know everything is okay. But, when you are sitting back in coach munching on stale peanuts crammed in a chair next to your stinky, snoring neighbor? This is the moment when the anxiety starts to creep back in. The disappearance of Malaysian Flight 370 also does not help matters. This mystery sent even the calmest of flyers into an anxiety-ridden psychological bend. Sure, we all know we can crash when we fly. We take that risk every time we board an airplane. But, we assume people will find us. We crash, we may die, but the authorities *will* find our bodies. Our families *will* be able to have a proper burial with whatever remains are left of us. But disappear on a commercial airliner? That's a problem. And, the disappearing commercial airliner scenario is something that was beyond our comprehension prior to MH370.

The other part of the story here is committing to a plan. Even if you have control, if you do not have a plan, that anxiety can creep right back in (Bunn, 2018). For instance, prior to boarding your aircraft, you may have been able to talk to your pilot before boarding, learning of his/her decades of experience, and even got to choose your seat. All of these pre-flight activities put you at ease, *because you feel in control*. But, what happens in an emergency? What happens if your bag won't fit in the overhead bin? What if someone is in your seat and refuses to move? All things that are real possibilities but are often not considered prior to boarding. Any of these things, without a plan, will tailspin you right back into your hole of despair.

There are things that passengers do to feel better. The quick fix is often prescription drugs. These drugs, such as Xanax and Valium, are sometimes prescribed to people with extreme flight anxiety. They make you so relaxed that even if the plane was crashing, you most likely would feel completely fine with it. Oh, and if you are under the influence, exiting the plane can be quite difficult when your body and psyche resemble that of a wet noodle. But, are these quick fixes really a good idea? These drugs treat anxiety, yes, but many times, these anxieties are a result of other anxieties (e.g., claustrophobia). In that case, these drugs won't *actually* treat your flight anxiety (Drillinger, 2018). But, just like when we feel out of control with our impending death, there are all-natural things we can do to help ourselves feel better when boarding a plane.

ALL-NATURAL WAYS OF CURBING FLIGHT ANXIETY

We already partake in many pre-flight activities that both lower our anxiety and serve death-denying functions. First, passengers will sometimes (read: rarely) listen to the safety message (or not). Listening to the safety message can provide a sense of comfort for passengers. By viewing the safety procedures, the passenger feels more in control. They are reminded that if they follow what is prescribed in the safety video, they can survive an air emergency or at least have a fighting chance. On the other hand, *not* listening to the safety message may also be helpful. And, based on my own anecdotal evidence and research by Lancaster et al. (2016), this seems to be the option most passengers choose. A safety message puts a death reminder straight in the face of an already anxious airline passenger. Ignoring the message is *exactly* what TMT would predict, a proximal response to a death reminder. What is ironic about this, though, is that by ignoring the safety message, you are actually at greater risk for death if an air emergency were to occur. For instance, it is hard to forget the stories that came out of the Hudson River crash-landing where passengers inflated their life vest while still in the aircraft, which resulted in a very difficult escape from the plane. Clearly, the message that life vests help you *float* failed these passengers. Perhaps if they would have listened to the safety message, that reminder would have stuck with them during their emergency.

Second, earbuds. We see all types of devices that passengers put over their ears in an attempt to forget where they are. Some listen to music, audiobooks, and some simply put them on so others will not talk to them (guilty as charged). All of this reduces anxiety because the earbuds give you a sense of comfort, whether that comfort comes from what you are listening to or simply the comfort that strangers will not try to engage you in conversation.

Third, pre-flight seat selection. Talk to any aviation expert and they will all agree: seat selection matters in a crash. When a plane crashes, the front of the plane experiences the largest amount of g-forces while the back of the place experiences the least. And, on a controlled crash-landing, such as Turkish Airlines Flight 1952 did when landing in Amsterdam in February 2009, the aircraft typically breaks into three distinct pieces, and in roughly the same places, depending on aircraft. I do not think I have to tell you (but I'm going to anyway) how unfortunate it would be to sit in the row where the plane broke. Life altering, in fact. Seat selection matters.

While we already engage in pre-flight anxiety-reducing behaviors, there still remains a fair amount of uncertainty. Therefore, there is more we can do to feel safe and to help curb some of that pesky anxiety that loves to appear once we've settled into our seat in 6B. There are some additional things that passengers can do in the days leading up to a flight, as well as on the day of the flight, that can seriously lower the potential for anxiety while in flight. While this is not an exhaustive list, taking even just one of these measures would be a good idea, because don't you want to be as relaxed as possible for the flight? I do (table 8.1).

First, limit aviation disaster–related media. As much as a week before your flight, consider limiting air-disaster media. Do not scour the interwebs for stories about your airline, aircraft, or search for recent air emergencies. Searching for these stories might be tempting, after all knowing is surely going to feel better, right? *Wrong*. Don't do it. Try to avoid movies with air emergencies like *Flight*. Great movie, terrifying crash sequence. Even if the movie is satire, such as *Airplane*, little seeds of doubt are still planted, and you will be surprised how easily those memories come to mind once you find yourself on the plane. Interested in MH370? Now is not the time to explore that interest. I can even assure you that no part of this book was written on an airplane.

Second, fill your carry-on with things that give you comfort, and keep those things easy to access in an organized travel bag that will fit under the seat in front of you. Dig into that bag the moment you settle in your seat. Indulge in that magazine you have not had time to read. Watch something

Table 8.1 Suggestions for the Flying Public

1. Limit aviation disaster–related media.
2. Fill your carry-on with things that give you comfort and joy.
3. Rely on flight anxiety apps.
4. Avoid alcohol and antianxiety prescription medications.

enticing on Netflix (non-airplane related, of course). Pack your own travel blanket (I own a very compact one purchased from The Container Store that gives me great joy). Play Candy Crush. Whatever makes you relaxed and happy, do that immediately. While this keeps you relaxed and happy, it also serves as a nice distraction for your psyche.

Third, rely on applications like "Am I Going Down?" to help you realize crashes are extremely rare. Okay, I know what you are thinking. Just the name of this application is frightening. Maybe, but plane crashes *are* rare. And, this application prides itself as a fear of flying application. Created in 2015, this application is "designed to reassure and empower those with a fear of flying" (N.A., 2000). You simply put in your airline, type of aircraft, and route and the application will tell you the chance of crash and how many days it would take for a crash to occur if you flew that route every day. Here's a hint: it is going to be an incredibly small chance, so theoretically you should feel much better. For instance, *New York Times* journalist Ondine Cohane said this about the application: "I could fly this route once a day for 14,000 years safely! The bumps started to feel less catastrophic. I eased my grip on the armrest" (N.A., 2020).

Fourth, avoid alcohol and prescription drugs if you can. There are some people that have severe cases of aviophobia. These people need the prescription drugs. In this case, the plane is actually safer when the prescription drugs are taken. But, these situations are rare. Furthermore, many of the less severe cases may turn to alcohol to mend their fears. Look, alcohol is *not* the answer to relaxing in flight. Not even a little bit. Not only does it dehydrate you (something flying already does a pretty good job of) but being inebriated also doesn't put you in a good position during or after flight. For instance, during flight you might get too rowdy and do something that has legal repercussions. And, describing lost luggage or attempting to find your hotel seems to be much more difficult in a foreign location while drunk.

We need a healthier flying public. By eliminating stressors and keeping our anxieties in check, we can avoid a multitude of potential unsavory situations. Like Alberto Brandi-Rivera when he had an outburst at the gate, violently knocking down signs, taking off his clothes, and getting in the faces of passengers at Charlotte Douglas International Airport. Note that the gate he was at was not the gate of his departing flight. You wouldn't want to be like Chloe Haynes who threatened to kill everyone on board a Jet2 flight and attempted to open the emergency door while in flight. Haynes was highly intoxicated at the time of this incident. Last, Anila Daulatzia had an outburst on her Southwest flight before even leaving the ground because there were dogs on the plane. She had to be physically lifted off the plane by local authorities after refusing to leave. All three of these incidents involved jail time consequences. And, these are merely just an example. Incidents like these are happening at an alarming frequency. All of these incidents (and the media coverage of them) have the potential to ignite flight anxiety in even the calmest of flyers. TMT argues that we can buffer this anxiety. We can do this by focusing on the hard and true fact that the likelihood of death by way of plane crash is statistically small. By focusing on that, rather than the high-profile plane crashes, we as a flying public can attempt to keep our anxieties in check and have a healthier flying experience for all.

References

Adelson, J., Simerman, J., & Calder, C. (2019, November 6). No turbulence and rave reviews so far for New Orleans' new airport terminal. Retrieved from: https://www.nola.com/ news/business/article_92c626c4-00bb011ea-aa6c-275e7c1009cc.html.

Adler, A. (1930). *Understanding Human Nature*. New York: Greenberg.

Agroskin, D. & Jonas, E. (2013). Controlling death by defending ingroups – Mediational insights in to terror management and control restoration. *Journal of Experimental Social Psychology, 49,* 1144–58. http://dx.doi.org/10.1016/j.jesp.2013.05.014.

Ahmad, I. (2014). World-class airport for a world-class city. *Journal of Airport Management, 8(3),* 206–13.

Alexander, I.E., Colley, R.S., & Adlerstein, A.M. (1957). Is death a matter of indifference? *Journal of Psychology, 43,* 277.

American Psychiatric Association (2013). *Diagnostic and Statistical Manual of Mental Disorders* (5th ed.). Arlington, VA: Author.

Anderson, H.G. (1919). *The Psychology of Aviation. The Medical and Surgical Aspects of Aviation.* London: Oxford University Press.

Anxiety and Depression Association of America (2018). Social anxiety disorder. Retrieved from: https://adaa.org/understanding-anxiety/social-anxiety-disorder.

Azmi, M.N.L., Rahman, N.A.A.A., Halim, Z.A., & Hamid, M.F.A. (2016). Crisis management in communication: A study on MH370, MH17, and QZ8501 aviation tragedies. *Media Watch, 7(3),* 281–98. doi: 10.15655/mw/2016/v7i3/48555.

Baker, S. (2019, May 19). Boeing's response to the 737 max crisis confused and frightened people, making it hard to believe its apologies, experts say. Retrieved from: https://www.businessinsider.com/title.

Ball-Rokeach, S.J., & DeFleur, M.L. (1976). A dependency model of mass-media effects. *Communication Research, 3(1)*, 3–21. doi: https://doi.org/10,1177/009365027600300101.

Balslev, T., DeGrave, W.S., Muijtjens, A.M.M., & Scherpbier, A.J.J.A. (2005). Comparison of text and video cases in a postgraduate problema-based learning format. *Medical Education, 39(11)*, 1086–92. doi: 10.1111/j.1365-2929.2005.02314.x.

Batrawy, A. (2019, July 8). The first major airline just dropped Boeing's 737 max for a rival plane. Retrieved from: https://time.com/5622194/boeing-737-max-flyadeal-airbus/.

Becker, E. (1962). *The Birth and Death of Meaning*. New York: Free Press.

Becker, E. (1974). *The Denial of Death*. New York, NY: Simon & Schuster.

Becker, E. (1975). *Escape from Evil*. New York: Free Press.

Beckerling, L. (1997). Changi grows to meet passenger and cargo demands. *Business Review Weekly, 19(22)*, 102.

Bier, L.M., Park, S., & Palenchar, M. (2018). Framing the flight MH370 mystery: A content analysis of Malaysian, Chinese, & U.S. Media. *International Communication Gazette, 80(2)*, 158–84. doi: 10.1177/1748048517707440.

Bodas, M., Siman-Tov, M., Peleg, K., & Solomon, Z. (2015). Anxiety-inducing media: The effect of constant news broadcasting on the well-being of Israeli television viewers. *Psychiatry: Interpersonal & Biological Processes, 78(3)*, 265–76. doi: 10.1080/00332747.

Boman, K., Lindahl, A., & Björk, O. (2003). Disease-related distress in parents of children with cancer at various stages after the time of diagnosis. *Acta Oncologica, 42(2)*, 137–46. doi: 10.1080/02841860310004995.

Bond, D.C. (1952). *The Love and Fear of Flying*. New York, NY: The International University Press.

Bor, R. (2007). Psychological factors in airline passenger and crew behavior: A clinical overview. *Travel Medicine and Infectious Diseases, 5*, 207–16. doi: http://dx.doi.org/10.1016/j.tmaid.2007.03.003.

Boyar, J.I. (1964). The construction and partial validation of a scale for the measurement of the fear of death. *Dissertation Abstracts, 25*, 20–1.

Bryant, A. (1994). USAir must now combat fliers' fears. *New York Times, 143(49815)*, 9.

Bunn, T. (2018). Pre-flight anxiety: What causes it, what stops it. Retrieved from: https://www.psychologytoday.com/us/blog/conquer-fear-flying/201807/pre-flight- anxiety-what-causes-it-what-stops-it

Burke, B.L., Kosloff, S., & Landau, M.J. (2013). Death goes to the polls: A meta-analysis of mortality salience effects on political attitudes. *Political Psychology, 34(2)*, 183–200. doi: https://doi.org.10.1111/pops.12005.

Burke, B.L., Martens, A., & Faucher, E.H. (2010). Two decades of terror management theory: A meta-analysis of mortality salience research. *Personality Social Psychological Review, 14*, 155–95. doi: 10.1177/1088868309352321.

Bushman, B.J. (1998). Effects of warning and information labels on consumption of full-fat, reduced-fat, and no-fat products. *Journal of Applied Psychology, 83*, 97–101. doi: 10.1037//0021-9010.83.1.97.

Busscher, B., & Spinhoven, P. (2017). Cognitive coping as a mechanism of change in cognitive- behavioral therapy for fear of flying: A longitudinal study with three-year follow-up. *Journal of Clinical Psychology, 73(9)*, 1064–75. doi: 10.1002/jclp.22424.

Butcher, J.N., & Hatcher, C. (1988). The neglected entity in air disaster planning: Psychological Services. *American Psychologist, 43(9),* 724–9.

Byrne, M.E., Shomaker, L.B., Brady, S.M., Kozlosky, M., Yanovski, J.A., & Tanofsky-Kraff, M. (2020). Association between latent trait negative affect and patterns of food-intake among girls with loss-of-control eating. *International Journal of Eating Disorders, 53(4),* 618–24. doi: 10.1002/eat.23253.

Capetillo-Ventura, N., & Juárez-Trevino, M. (2015). Internet addiction in university medical students. *Medicina Universitaria, 17(67),* 88–93. doi: 10.1016/j.rmu.2015.02.003.

Carbonell, D. (2019, May 17). What causes fear of flying? Retrieved from: https://www.anxietycoach.com/causes-fear-of-flying.html.

Cartledge, M. (2016, July). The world's best airport? *Aviation News: The Past, Present, and Future of Flight,* 62–7.

Cheng, J.W., Hitomo, H., Otsuka, T., & Jean, S.Y. (2016). Cultivation effects of mass and social media on perceptions and behavioral intentions in post-disaster recovery – The case of the 2011 Great East Japan Earthquake. *Telematics and Informatics, 33*(3), 753–72. doi: 10.1016/j.tele.2015.12.001.

Changsong, W., Yiming, C., & Ahmad, J.H. (2017). A comparative study of social media users' perception on the Malaysia Airlines flight MH370 incident in mainland China and Malaysia. *International Journal of Culture and History, 3(2),* 1–23. doi: 10.18178/ijch.2017.3.2.091.

Chant, D. (2015). Planning small and medium-sized airports for flexibility and future growth. *Journal of Airport Management, 9(3),* 223–31.

Collimore, K.C., McCabe, R.E., Carleton, R.N., & Asmundson, G.J.G. (2008). Media exposure and dimensions of anxiety sensitivity: Differential associations with PTSD symptom clusters. *Journal of Anxiety Disorders, 22(6),* 1021–8.

Correa, C. (2019, September 4). Designing an airport to be more than just a gateway. Retrieved from: https://www.internationalairportreview.com/article/102079/design-construction- jewel-changi-airport/.

Cowley, G. (2017, July 18). Fear of flying (Aviophobia): How to defeat it. Retrieved from: https://www.medicalnewstoday.com/articles/100609.php.

Cui, D., & Wu, F. (2017). Inter-media agenda setting in global news production: Examining agenda attributes in newspaper coverage of the MH370 incident in the U.S., China, and Hong Kong. *Asian Journal of Communication, 27(6),* 582–600. doi: https://doi.org/10/1080/01292986.2017.1305426.

Davies, N. (2018). *Beneath Another Sky: A Global Journey into History.* Allen Lane.

Davis, D. (2019). Flight anxiety statistics. Retrieved from: https://flyfright.com/statistics.

Department of Homeland Security (2017). Written testimony of CBP Paul Beeson, Director of DHS Joint Task Force – West for a House Committee on Homeland Security, Subcommitee on border and maritime security hearing titled, "A dangerous and sophisticated advisory: The threat to the homeland posed by cartel operations." Retrieved from: https://www.dhs.gov/news/2017/02/16/written-testimony-cbp-house-homeland-security-subcommittee-border-and-maritime.

Drillinger, M. (2018). Xanax to Booze: What doctors really think about your in-flight anti- anxiety tricks. Retrieved from: https://www.healthline.com/health/mental-health/worst- flight-anxiety-tricks-healthy-tips

de Neufville, R., & Odoni, A.R. (2003). *'Airport Systems: Planning, Design, & Management'*. McGraw Hill: New York.

Ducharme, J. (2018, July 6). Why some people have a crippling fear of flying – And how they can overcome it. Retrieved from: https://time.com/5330978/fear-of-flying-aviophobia/.

Edwards, B. (2005). *The Modern Airport Terminal* (2nd ed.). London and New York: Spon Press.

Ekeberg, ø., Fauske, B., & Berg-Hansen, B. (2014). Norwegian airline passengers are not more afraid of flying after the terror act of September 11. The flight anxiety, however, is significantly attributed to acts of terrorism. *Scandinavian Journal of Psychology, 55,* 464–8.

Farhi, P. (2018, March 20). How breaking news got panelized: On cable, journalists and pundits increasingly share space. *The Washington Post.*

Federal Aviation Administration (2019). Passengers & Cargo: Unruly passengers. Retrieved from: https://www.faa.gov/data_research/passengers_cargo/unruly_passengers/.

Ferrer, R., & Klein, W.M. (2015). Risk perceptions and health behavior. *Current Opinions in Psychology, 5,* 85–9. doi: 10.106/j.copsyc.2015.03.012.

Ford, D. (2014). Why are we so gripped by missing Malaysia Airlines Flight 370? Retrieved from: https://www.cnn.com/2014/03/17/world/asia/malaysia-airlines-plane-fascination/index.html.

Fox News. (2018, December 21). Most bizarre airline incidents of 2018. Retrieved from: https://www.foxnews.com/travel/most-bizarre-airline-incidents-of-2018.

Fransen, M.L., Smeesters, D., & Fennis, B.M. (2011). The role of social presence in mortality salience effects. *Journal of Business Research, 64*, 29–33. doi: 10.1016/j.jbusres.2009.09.016.

French, J.R.P. (1968). The conceptualization and measurement of mental health in terms of self-identity theory. In S.B. Bells (Ed.), *The Definition and Measurement of Mental Health.* Washington, D.C.: U.S. Department of Health, Education, and Welfare.

Freud, S. (1936). *The Problem of Anxiety.* Psychoanalytic Quarterly Press.

Fukada, H. (1986). Psychological processes mediating persuasion-inhibiting effect of forewarning in fear-arousing communication. *Psychology Reports, 58,* 87–90. doi: 10.2466/pr0.1986.58.1.87.

Galovski, T.E., Blain, L.M., Chappuis, C., & Fletcher, T. (2013). Sex differences in recovery from PTSD in male and female interpersonal assault survivors. *Behaviour Research & Therapy, 51(6),* 247–55. https://doi.org/10.1016/j.brat.2013.02.002.

Garrett, R.K., Weeks, B.E., & Neo, R.L. (2016). Driving a wedge between evidence and beliefs: How online ideological news exposure promotes political misperceptions. *Journal of Computer-Mediated Communication, 21,* 331–48. doi: 10.111/jcc4.12164.

Gerber, Z. & Anaki, D. (2019). Self-compassion as a buffer against concrete but not abstract threat. *Death Studies, 43(10),* 639–46. doi: 10.1080/07481187.2018.1511195.

Gerbner, G., Gross, L., Morgan, M., & Signorielli, N. (1980). The "mainstreaming" of America: Violence profile no. 11. *Journal of Communication, 30,* 10–29.

Glisson, L. (2019). Breaking the spin cycle: Teaching complexity in the age of fake news. *Portal: Libraries and the Academy, 19(3),* 461–84. doi: 10.1353/pla.2019.0027.

Golson, J. (2015). The most logical (and craziest) MH370 conspiracy theories. Retrieved from: https://www.wired.com/2015/03/logical-craziest-mh370-conspiracy- theories/.

Gonzales, L. (2014). *Flight 232: A Story of Disaster and Survival.* New York, NY: Norton.

Greenberg, J., Solomon, S., & Pyszczynski, T. (1997). Terror management theory of self- esteem and cultural worldviews and empirical assessments and conceptual refinements. In M. Zana's (Ed.), *Advances in Experimental Psychology.* Orlando, FL: Academic Press.

Greenberg, J., Pyszczynski, T., & Solomon, S. (1986). The causes and consequences of a need for self-esteem: A terror management theory. In R.F. Baumeister's (Ed.), *Public Self & Private Self* (pp. 189–212). Springer Series in Social Psychology.

Greenberg, J., Pyszczynski, T., Solomon, S., Pinel, E., Simon, L., & Jordan, K. (1993). Effects of self-esteem on vulnerability-denying defensive distortions: Further evidence of an anxiety-buffering function of self-esteem. *Journal of Experimental Social Psychology, 29,* 229–51. doi: 10/1006/jesp.1993.1010.

Greenberg, J., Solomon, S., Pyszczynski, T., Rosenblatt, A., Burling, J., Lyon, D., & Simon, L. (1992). Assessing the terror management analysis of self-esteem: Converging evidence of an anxiety-buffering function. *Journal of Personality & Social Psychology, 63,* 913–22.

Greenberg, J., Pyszczynski, T., Solomon, S., Rosenblatt, A., Veeder, M., Kirkland, S., & Lyon, D. (1990). Evidence for terror management theory II: The effects of mortality salience on reactions to those who threaten or bolster the cultural worldview. *Journal of Personality and Social Psychology, 58(2),* 308–18.

Greenberg, J., Simon, L., Pyszczynski, T., Solomon, S., & Chatel, D. (1992). Terror management and tolerance: does mortality salience always intensify negative reactions to others who threaten one's worldview? *Journal of Personality and Social Psychology, 63,* 212–20. doi: 10.1037//0022-3514.63.2.212.

Greer, C.F., & Moreland, K.D. (2003). United airlines' and American airlines' online crisis communication following the September 11 terrorist attacks. *Public Relations Review, 29(4),* 427–42. doi: 10.1016/j.pubrev.2003.08.005.

Halim, R. (2014). From KL to Beijing: MH370, the media and the meaning of a disaster. *Procedia-Social & Behavioral Sciences, 155,* 171–7. doi: 10.1016/j.sbspro.2014.10.275.

Harmon-Jones, E., Simon, L., Greenberg, J., Pyszczynski, T., Solomon, S., & McGregor, H. (1997). Terror management theory and self-esteem: Evidence that increased self-esteem reduces mortality salience efforts. *Journal of Personality and Social Psychology, 72,* 24–36.

Harvell, L.A. (2016). Death or social exclusion? An exploration of social isolation and religious affiliation. Presented at the annual meeting of the Eastern Communication Association in Baltimore, Maryland.

Harvell, L.H., Nisbett, G.S., Wong, N.C.H., & McCloskey, Y. (2013, April). Apocalyptic Doom: How religion and mortality salience affect fears of the 2012 Mayan Prophecy. Presented at the annual meeting of the Central States Communication Association in Kansas City, MO.

Harvell-Bowman, L.A., Critchfield, K.L., Ndzana, F., Stucker, E., Wilgus, K., Hurst, A., & Sullivan, K. (2020, February). Of love and death: Death anxiety, attachment, and suicide as experienced by college students. Presented at the annual meeting of the Society for Personality and Social Psychology in New Orleans, LA.

Harvell, L.A. & Nisbett, G.A. (2016). *Denying Death: An Interdisciplinary Approach to Terror Management Theory.* London, UK: Routledge.

Harvell, L.A., Stillman, T., Nisbett, G.S., Cranney, K., & Schow, A. (2016). A field investigation of flight anxiety: Evidence of gender differences in consumer behaviors among Las Vegas passengers. *Journal of Airline and Airport Management, 6(1),* 2014–4806. doi: http://dx.doi.org/10.3926.jairm.41.

Hemmerdinger, J. (2019). FAA 2018 analysis warned of 15 fatal MAX crashes months before second accident. *Flightglobal.*

Hetsroni, A., & Tukachinsky, R.H. (2006). Television-world estimates, real-world estimates, and television viewing: A new scheme for cultivation. *Journal of Communication, 56,* 133–56.

Higgins, E. (2019). *The Hunt for MH370.* Australia: Pan MacMillan.

Hmielowski, J., Beam, M., & Hutchens, M. (2015). Structural changes in media and attitude polarization: Examining the contribution of television news before and after the Telecommunications Act of 1996. *International Journal of Public Opinion Research, 28,* 153–72. doi: 10.1093/ijpor/edv012.

Hohman, Z.P. & Hogg, M.A. (2015). Mortality salience, self-esteem, and defense of the group: Mediating role of in-group identification. *Journal of Applied Social Psychology, 45,* 80–9. doi: 10.1111/jasp.12277.

Hoopfer, E. (2018, November 19). Transcript details what happened aboard fatal Southwest flight. Retrieved from: https://www.bizjournals.com/dallas/news/2018/11/19/title.

Horney, K. (1937). *The Neurotic Personality of Our Time.* New York: Psychology Press.

Houston, J.B. (2009). Media coverage of terrorism: A meta-analytic assessment of media use and posttraumatic stress. *Journalism & Mass Communication Quarterly, 86(4)*, 844–61.

IATA (2019). Unruly passengers. Retrieved from: https://www.iata.org/en/policy/consumer-pax-rights/unruly-passengers.

Irwin, R.E. (2020). Misinformation and de-contextualization: International media reporting on Sweden and COVID-19. *Globalization & Health, 16(1),* 1–12.

James, W. (1890). *The Principles of Psychology.* Courier Corporation.

Joiner, T.E. (2007). *Why People Die by Suicide.* Cambridge, MA: Harvard University Press.

Josephs, L. (2018, August 13). 'Incredible maneuvers' by airline ground agent who stole plane baffles employer. His only training appears to be 'video games'. Retrieved from: https://www.cnbc.com/2018/08/13.

Kim, E., Shepherd, M.E., & Clinton, J.D. (2020). The effect of big-city news on rural America during the COVID-19 pandemic. *Proceedings of the National Academy of Sciences of the United States of America, 117(36),* 1–6.

Klein, J. (2019). Perils and promise in the modern media industry. *Brown Journal of World Affairs, 25(2),* 211–21.

Klein Tuente, S., Bogaerts, S., & Veling, W. (2019). Hostile attribution bias and aggression in adults – A systematic review. *Aggression & Violent Behavior, 46,* 66–81. doi: 10.1016/j.avb.2019.01.009.

Kleinert, J. (2002). An approach to sport injury trait anxiety: Scale construction and structure analysis. *European Journal of Sport Science, 2(3),* 1–12. doi: 10.1080/17461390200072305.

Kosloff, S., Anderson, G., Nottbohm, A., & Hoshiko, B. (2019). Proximal and distal terror management defenses: A systematic review and analysis. In C. Routledge & M. Vess's (Eds.), *Handbook of Terror Management Theory* (pp. 31–64). London, UK: Elsevier. doi: https://doi.org/10.1016/B978-0-12-811844-3.00002-0.

Kraaij, V., Garnefski, N., & Van Gerwen, L. (2003). Cognitive coping and anxiety symptoms among people who seek help for fear of flying. *Aviation, Space, and Environmental Medicine, 74(3),* 273–7.

Kubany, E.S., Abueg, F.R., Owens, J.A., Brennan, J.M., Kaplan, A.S., & Watson, S.B. (1995). Initial examination of a multidimensional model of trauma-related guilt: Applications to combat veterans and battered women. *Journal of Psychopathology & Behavioral Assessment, 17,* 353–76.

Laker, M. (2012). Specific phobia: Flight. *Activitas Nervosa Superior, 54,* 3–4.

Lancaster, A., Bowman, N.D., & Harvell, L.A. (2015, November). Flying blind to safety: Mortality salience, efficacy, and message recall of airline safety demonstrations. Presented at the annual meeting of the National Communication Association in Las Vegas, NV.

Lancaster, A.L., Bowman, N.D., & Harvell, L.A. (2016). "Death is coming, but I'm too scared to think about it": Defining and distinguishing the roles of death and fear as motivators to cognitive, affective, and behavioral change. In L.A. Harvell & G.S. Nisbett's (Eds.), *Denying Death: An Interdisciplinary Approach to Terror Management Theory* (pp. 136–49). Oxford, UK: Routledge.

Landreville, K.D., & Niles, C. (2019). "And that's a fact!": The roles of political ideology, PSRs, and perceived source credibility in estimating factual content in partisan news. *Journal of Broadcasting & Electronic Media, 63(2),* 177–94. doi: 10.1080/08838151.2019.1622339.

Leigh, G. (2019, November 13). New Orleans' ambitious new airport is open, but does it measure up? Retrieved from: https://www.forbes.com/sites/gabrielleigh/2019/11/13/new-orleans-ambitious-new-airport-is-open-but-does-it-measure-up/#5debe8ac4422.

Lemal, M., & Van den Bulck, J. (2011). Television news coverage about cervical cancer: Impact on female viewers' vulnerability perceptions and fear. *European Journal of Public Health, 21(3),* 381–6. doi: 10.1093/eurpub/ckq040.

Limer, E. (2019, March 27). Lion Air pilots had less than a minute to avert fatal crash. Retrieved from: https://www.popularmechanics.com/flight/airlines/a26962587.

Lowinger, T., & Solomon, Z. (2004). PTSD, guilt, and shame among reckless drivers. *Journal of Loss & Trauma, 9,* 327–44. doi: 10.1080/15325020490477704.

Martin, I.M., & Kamins, M.A. (2010). An application of terror management theory in the design of social and health-related anti-smoking appeals. *Journal of Consumer Behaviour, 9,* 172–90. doi: 10.1002/cb.293.

Martyn, P., & Brymer, E. (2016). The relationship between nature relatedness and anxiety. *Journal of Health Psychology, 21(7),* 1436–45. doi: 10.1177/1359105314555169.

Masunaga, S. (2019). How the design of Boeing's 737 Max cost CEO Muilenburg his job. Retrieved from: https://www.latimes.com/business/story/2019-12-23/boeing- 737-max-dennis-muilenburg

Medvedev, A., Alomar, I., & Augustyn, S. (2017). Innovation in airport design. *Aviation, 21(1),* 23–8. doi: 10.3846/16487788.2017.1303542.

Mestre, C., Lopes, A., Reis, C., Lemos de Costa, S., & Albuquerque, C. (2017). Translation and validation of two questionnaires assessing fear of flying for Portuguese language. *Análise Psicológica, 3(XXXV)*, 367–81. doi: 10.14417/ap.1197.

Minkel, S. (2009). Communication during a crisis. Retrieved from: https://platformmagazine.org/2009/02/25/communication-during-a-crisis/.

Mintz, Z. (2014). MH17 crisis response: Has Malaysia Airlines learned from MH370 disaster? Retrieved from: https://www.ibtimes.com/mh17-crisis-response-has- malaysia-airlines-learned-mh370-disaster-1631690

Mo Bahk, C. (2006). College students' perceived risk and anxiety after reading airplane crash news. *Psychological Reports, 99(1),* 107–10. doi: 10.2466/PRO.99.1.107–10.

Moon, H.G. (2019). Mindfulness of death as a tool for mortality salience induction with reference to terror management theory. *Religions, 10(6)*, 353. doi: 10.3390/rel10060353.

Mühlberger, A., Weik, A., Pauli, P., & Weidemann, G. (2006). One-session virtual reality exposure treatment for fear of flying: One-year follow-up and graduation flight accompaniment effects. *Psychotherapy Research, 16,* 26–40.

Murphy, G. (1947). *Personality.* New York: Harper.

Nabi, R.L., & Prestin, A. (2016). Unrealistic hope and unnecessary fear: Exploring how sensationalistic news stories influence health behavior motivation. *Health Communication.* doi: 10.1080/10410236.2015.1045237.

Nacoste, R.W., & Hummels, B. (1994). Affirmative action and the behavior of decision makers. *Journal of Applied Social Psychology, 24,* 595–613.

Nail, P.R. & McGregor, I. (2009). Conservative shift among liberals and conservatives following 9/11/01. *Social Justice Research, 22(2–3),* 231–40. doi: https://doi.org/10.1007/s11211-009-0098-x.

Naveh-Kedem, Y. & Sverdlik, N. (2019). Changing prosocial values following an existential threat as a function of political orientation: Understanding the effects of armed conflicts from a terror management perspective. *Personality & Individual Differences,* 150. doi: 10.1016/j.paid.2019.07.004.

Nisbett, G.S., & Harvell, L.H. (2013, March). Anxiety and politics: Applying terror management theory to political decisions. Presented at the mid-winter meeting of the Association for Education in Journalism and Mass Communication in Norman, OK.

No Author. (2019). Estimated June 2019 U.S. Airline Traffic Data. Retrieved from: https://www.bts.gov/newsroom/estimated-june-2019-us-airline-traffic-data#:~:text=For%20the%20first%20half%20of,and%20up%2011.5%25%20from%2020 16.

No Author. (2019). How can you cope with fear of flying? Retrieved from: https://www..medicalnewstoday.com/articles/320367.php#1.

No Author. (2020). Retrieved from: https://www.fearsofflying.app.

No Author. (2020). American Psychological Association Dictionary. Retrieved from: https://dictionary.apa.org

No Author. (2020). CNN launches. Retrieved from: https://www.history.com/this-day- in-history/cnn-launches.

No Author. (2019). This is what makes us the most stressed at airports. Retrieved from: https://www.prioritypass.com/en/blog/2019/airport-stress-survey.

Nousi, A., van Gerwen, L., & Spinhoven, P. (2008). The flight anxiety situations questionnaire and the flight anxiety modality questionnaire: Norms for people with fear of flying. *Travel Medicine and Infectious Disease, 6,* 305–10. doi: 10.1016/j.tmaid.2008.06.001.

Oakes, M. & Bor, R. (2010). The psychology of fear of flying (Part I): A critical evaluation of current perspectives on the natures, prevalence, and etiology of fear of flying. *Travel Medicine & Infectious Disease, 8,* 327–38. doi: http://dx.doi.org/10.1016/j.tmaid.2010.10.

Padgett, J., Dunaway, J., & Darr, J.P. (2019). As seen on TV? How gatekeeping makes the U.S. House seem more extreme. *Journal of Communication, 69(6),* 696–719. doi: 10.1093/joc/jqz039.

Paek, H.J., Oh, S.H., & Hove, T. (2016). How fear-arousing news messages affect risk perceptions and intention to talk about risk. *Health Communication.* doi: 10.1080/10410236.2015.1037419.

Park, S., Bier, M., & Palenchar, M.J. (2016). Framing a mystery: Information subsidies and media coverage of Malaysia airlines flight 370. *Public Relations Review,* 42(4), 654–64. doi: 10.1016/j.pubrev.2016.06.004.

Park, Y-C. & Pyszczynski, T. (2019). Reducing defensive responses to thoughts of death: Meditation, mindfulness, and Buddhism. *Journal of Personality & Social Psychology, 116(1),* 101–18. doi: 10.1037/pspp0000163.

Paul, K. (2018). FAA declines to put a stop to the 'incredible shrinking airline seat'. Retrieved from: https://www.marketwatch.com/story/faa-declines-to-put-a-stop-to-the-incredible- shrinking-airline-seat-2018-07-09.

Perloff, R.M. (2014). *The Dynamics of Political Communication: Media & Politics in a digital age.* New York, NY: Routledge.

Plusnin, N., Pepping, C.A., & Kashima, E.S. (2018). The role of close relationships in terror management: A systematic review and research agenda. *Personality & Social Psychology, 22(4),* 307–46. doi: 10.1177/1088868317753505.

Post, N.M. (2019, June 24). Where's the mall? Complex constructed forest hiding Singapore Airport's shopping center demanded compromise. *Engineering News-Record,* 30–7.

Pujol, R. (2014). Malaysia Airlines disappearance joins greatest mysteries of all time. Retrieved from: https://pixll.com/2014/03/17/Malaysia-airlines-disappear-ance-joins-greatest- mysteries-of-all-time/.

Pyszczynski, T., Greenberg, J., & Solomon, S. (1999). A dual-process model of defense against conscious and unconscious death-related thoughts: An extension of terror management theory. *Psychological Review, 106(4),* 835–45. doi: 10.1037//0033-295X.106.4.835.

Pyszczynski, T., Wicklund, R.A., Floresku, S., Koch, H., Gauch, G., Solomon, S., & Greenberg, J. (1996). Whistling in the dark: Exaggerated consensus estimates in response to incidental reminders of mortality. *Psychological Science, 7*(6), 332–6. doi: 10.1111/j.1967-9280.1996.tb00384.x.

Quest, R. (2016). *The Vanishing Flight MH370: The True Story of the Hunt for the Missing Malaysian Plane.* Berkley: Penguin.

Rank, O. (1950). *Psychology and the Soul.* New York: A.S. Barnes & Co..

Reed, T. (2015). Twenty-five years ago, U.S. airlines banned smoking on domestic flights. Retrieved from: https://www.forbes.com/sites/tedreed/2015 /02/24/twenty-five-years- ago-U-S-airlines-banned-smoking-on-domestic-flights/#350341925407.

Rivers, D. (2019). MH370 pilot was 'in toilet when plane depressurised' causing jet to CRASH. Retrieved from: https://www.dailystar.co.uk/news/world-news/mh370 -news- pilot-toilet-crash-16830329.

Robson, M. (2020). The most stressful job in the world? What it's really like to be an air traffic controller. Retrieved from: https://www .forbes.com/sites/michelerobson/2020/05/29/the-most-stressful-job-in -the- world-what-its-really-like-to-be-an-air-traffic-controller/#47ccd7ac1c04.

Röderer, K., & Cervinka, R. (2012). Mental representations of nature – The importance of well-being. In S. Kabisch, A. Kunath, & R. Schweizer-Reis et al. (Eds.), *Vulnerability, Risks, & Complexity: Impacts of Global Change on Human Habitats (Advances in Environmental Studies), vol. 3* (pp. 243–54). Göttingen: Hogrefe Publishing.

Rogers, C.R. (1959). A theory of therapy, personality, and interpersonal relationships, as developed in the client-centered framework. In S. Koch (Ed.), *Psychology: A Study of a Science (Vol. 3).* New York: McGraw-Hill.

Rosenberg, M. (1965). *Society and the Adolescent Self-Image.* Princeton: Princeton University Press.

Rosenberg, M. & Simmons, R.G. (1972). *Black and white Self-Esteem: The Urban School Child.* Washington, DC: American Sociological Association.

Rosenblatt, A., Greenberg, J., Solomon, S., Pyszczynski, T., & Lyon, D. (1989). Evidence for Terror Management Theory: I. The effects of mortality salience on reactions to those who violate or uphold cultural values. *Journal of Personality & Social Psychology, 57(4),* 681–90.

Routledge, C. & Vess, M. (2019). *The Handbook of Terror Management Theory.* London, UK: Elsevier.

Rybalko, S. (2011). Russian disaster coverage is no accident: How two Russian newspapers and their readers frame a Russian plane crash. *Russian Journal of Communication, 4(1/2),* 53–71. doi: 10.1080/19409419.2011.10756790.

Sampath, H., Soohinda, G., Sharma, A., & Dutta, S. (2018). Media exposure to earthquake- related content in its aftermath as a risk factor for acute stress disorder. *Open Journal of Psychiatry & Allied Sciences, 9(2),* 152–6. doi: 10.595812394-2061.2018.0032.0.

Schaper, D. (2017). Despite viral incidents, passengers are more satisfied with airlines than ever. Retrieved from: https://npr.org/2017/05/16/528583117/despite-viral-incidents-passengers-are-more-satisfied-with-the-airlines-than-eve.

Schaper, D. (2020). FAA inches closer to approaching Boeing's fixes to troubled 737 Max. Retrieved from: https://www.npr.org/2020/07/21/893950168/faa-inches- closer-to-approving-boeings-fixes-to-troubled-737-max

Schindler, S., Reinhard, M-A., Dobiosch, S., Steffan-Fauseweh, I., Özdemir, G., & Greenberg, J. (2019). The attenuating effect of mortality salience on dishonest behavior. *Motivation & Emotion, 43(1),* 52–62. doi: 10.1007/s11031-018-9734-y.

Schults, D.M. & Arnow, R.C. (2019). Effects of a brief mindfulness induction on death-related anxiety. *Omega: Journal of Death and Dying, 79(3),* 313–35. doi: 10.1177/0030222817721115.

Self, W. (2014). Fearless flying is an act of collective delusion. If only you could still sit next to the pilot. *New Statesman, 143(5202),* 70.

Selk, A. (2018, February 18). Iran says fog caused a plane crash that may have killed 65. That might not be the whole story. Retrieved from: https://www.washington-post.com/news/ worldviews/wp/2018/02/18/title.

Sharkey, J. (2015, May 7). Bad flight? Well, there's the airport. *New York Times, F1.*

Sharma, B. (2019). Pilot in Nepal plane crash had 'emotional breakdown,' officials say. Retrieved from: https://www.nytimes.com/2019/01/28/world/asia/nepal-plane-crash- pilot.html.

Sherman, S.J., & Lynn, S.J. (1990). Social psychological principles in Milton Erickson's psychotherapy. *British Journal of Experimental and Clinical Hypnosis, 7,* 37–46.

Shuchi, S.N. (2016). A novel concept for airport terminal design integrating flexibility. *Queensland University of Technology.* Brisbane.

Shuchi, S., Drogemuller, R., & Buys, L. (2017). Flexibility in airport terminals: Identification of design factors. *Journal of Airport Management, 12(1),* 90–108.

Simon, L., Greenberg, J., Harmon-Jones, E., Solomon, S., Pyszczynski, T., Arndt, J., & Abend, T. (1997). Terror management and cognitive-experimental self-theory: evidence that terror management occurs in the experiential system. *Journal of Personality and Social Psychology, 72,* 1132–46.

Skapinakis, P., Bellos, S., Oikonomou, A., Dimitriadis, G., Gkikas, P., Perdikari, E., & Mavreas, V. (2020). Depression and its relationship with coping strategies and illness perceptions during the COVID-19 lockdown in Greece: A cross-sectional survey of the population. *Depression Research & Treatment,* 1–11.

Skolnick, R.B., Schare, M.L., Wyatt, K.P., & Tillman, M.A. (2012). Aviophobia Assessment: Validating the Flight Anxiety Situations Questionnaire as a clinical identification measure. *Journal of Anxiety Disorders, 26,* 779–84.

Slone, M., Shoshani, A., & Baumgarten-Katz, I. (2008). The relation between actual exposure to political violence and preparatory intervention for exposure to media coverage of terrorism. *Anxiety Stress Coping, 21(3),* 243–61. doi: 10.1080/10615800701510124.

Smith, K. (2019). Aerophobia: The fear of flying. Retrieved from: https://www.psycom.net/ aerophobia-fear-of-flying/.

Smith, M.B. (1978). Perspectives on selfhood. *American Psychologist, 33,* 1053–63.

Soenke, M., Cohen, F., Greenberg, J., & Lifshin, U. (2018). Are you smarter than a cetacean?: Death reminders and concerns about human intelligence. *Society & Animals, 26(5),* 469–89. doi: 10.1163/15685306-12341553.

Solomon, S., Greenberg, J., & Pyszczynski, T. (2015). *The Worm at the Core: On the Role of Death in Life.* New York, NY: Random House.

Sonnevent, J. (2018). Interruptions of time: the coverage of the missing Malaysian plane MH370 and the concept of 'events' in media research. *Journalism, 19(1),* 75–92. doi: https://doi.org/10.1177/1464884916680154.

Spinks, R. (2018a). Forget legroom – Air travelers are fed up with seat width. Retrieved from: https://qz.com/quartzy/1324754/airline-seats-are-getting-narrower-and-passengers-dont- like-it/.

Spinks, R. (2018b). Airlines have an alcohol problem – And some are blaming it on airports. Retrieved from: https://qz.com/quartzy/1311180/drinking-in-airports-airlines-are- cracking-down-on-alcohol-and-travel/.

Street, A.E., Gibson, L.E., & Holohan, D.R. (2005). Impact of childhood traumatic events, trauma-related guilt, and avoidant coping strategies on PTSD symptoms in female survivors of domestic violence. *Journal of Traumatic Stress, 18(3),* 245–52. https://doi.org/10.1002/jts.20026.

Street, F. (2019, December 3). Outrage in the skies: Are airline passengers getting more unruly? Retrieved from: https://www.cnn.com/travel/article/unruly-airplane-passengers/index.html.

Taubman Ben-Ari, O. (2000). The effect of reminders of death on reckless driving: A terror management perspective. *Current Directions in Psychological Science, 9(6),* 196–9. doi: 10.1080/07481180302898.

Taubman Ben-Ari, O., Florian, V., & Mikulincer, M. (1999). The impact of mortality salience on reckless driving: A test of terror management mechanisms. *Journal of Personality & Social Psychology, 76(1),* 35–45.

Templer, D.I. (1971). The relationship between verbalized and non-verbalized death anxiety. *Journal of Genetic Psychology, 119,* 211–14.

Terkel, A. (2020, Mar 25). The deadly consequences of Trump's attacks on the media in a pandemic. Retrieved from: https://www.huffpost.com/entry/trump-attack- media-coronavirus_n_5e790649c5b6f5b7c5491406.

The Week Staff (2020). What happened to the Malaysia Airlines Flight 370? Retrieved from: https://www.theweek.co.uk/mh370/58037/mh370-conspiracy-theories- what-happened-to-the-missing-plane.

U.S. Customs & Border Protection (2019). Office of Field Operations Nationwide Drug Seizures. Retrieved from: https://www.cbp.gov/newsroom/stats/cbp-enforcement-statistics-fy2019.

Vail, K.E., Courtney, E., & Arndt, J. (2019). The influence of existential threat and tolerance salience on anti-Islamic attitudes in American politics. *Political Psychology, 40(5)*, 1143–62. doi: 10.1111/pops.12579.

Vail, K.E., & Routledge, C. (2020). *The Science of Religion, Spirituality, & Existentialism.* London, UK: Elsevier.

Valinsky, J. (2019, July 17). United is buying used planes to add capacity as the 737 max remains grounded. Retrieved from: https://www.cnn.com/2019/07/17/business/title.

Van Gerwen, L.J., Diekstra, R.F., Arondeus, J.M., & Wolfger, R. (2004). Fear of flying treatment programs for passengers: An international update. *Aviation Space & Environmental Medicine, 2,* 27–35. doi: 10.1016/j.tmaid.2004.01.002.

Van Gerwen, L.J., Spinhoven, P., & Diekstra, R.F.W. (1999). Construction and psychometric characteristics of two self-reported questionnaires for the assessment of fear of flying. *Psychological Assessment, 11,* 146–58. doi: http://dx.doi.org/10.1037/1040- 3590.11.2.146.

Van Gerwen, L.J., Spinhoven, P., Dieckstra, R.F.W., & Van Dick, R. (1997). People who seek help for fear of flying: Typology of flying phobias. *Behavior Therapy, 28,* 237–51. doi: http://dx.doi.org/10.1016/S0005-7894(97)80045-7.

Van Orden, K.A., Witte, T.K., Cukrowicz, K.C., Braithwaite, S., Selby, E.A., & Joiner, T.E. (2010). The interpersonal theory of suicide. *Psychological Review, 117(2),* 575–600. doi: 10.1037/a0018697

Watts, J.M. (2014). Malaysia Airlines response to MH17 loss over Ukraine calmer than MH370. Retrieved from: https://www.wsj.com/articles/malaysia-airlines-response-to-mh17-loss- calmer-than-mh370-1405687116.

Weathersby Jr., W. (2003). Singapore's Changi Airport rail station transports travelers through multiple levels infused with light. *Architectural Record, 191(11),* 242–6.

Wen, J. (2020). Response to "a rejoinder to misleading articles about misleading media coverage: A case of COVID-19" by professor Stephen Pratt. *Anatolia: An International Journal of Tourism & Hospitality Research, 31(3)*, 519–21. doi: 10.1080/13032917.2020.1775000.

Wen, J., Aston, J., Liu, X., & Ying, T. (2020). Effects of misleading media coverage on public health crisis: A case of the 2019 novel coronavirus outbreak in China. *Anatolia: An International Journal of Tourism & Hospitality Research, 31(2),* 331–6.

Wilson, G. (2012). *Community Resilience and Environmental Transitions.* London: Routledge.

Winkler, R.C. & Myers, R.A. (1963). Some concomitants of self-ideal discrepancy measures of self-acceptance. *Journal of Counseling Psychology, 10,* 83–6.

Witte, K. (1994). Fear control and danger control: a test of the extended parallel process model (EPPM). *Communication Monographs, 61,* 113–34. doi: 10.1080/03637759409376328.

Witte, K., & Allen, M. (2000). A meta-analysis of fear appeals: Implications for effective public health campaigns. *Health Education & Behavior, 27(5),* 591–615. doi: https://doi.org/10.1177/109019810002700506.

Wong, N.C.H., Nisbett, G.S., & Harvell, L.A. (2016). Smoking is so ew! College smokers' reactions to health- vs. social-focused antismoking threat messages. *Health Communication.* doi: 10.1080/10410236.2016.1140264

Wormwood, J.B., Lin, Y-R., Lynn, S.K., Barrett, L.F., & Quigley, K.S. (2019). Psychological impact of mass violence depends on affective tone of media content. *PLoS ONE, 14(4),* 1–20. doi: 10.1371/journal.pone.0213891.

Wrigley, S. (2019). The reckless final approach of US Bangla Flight 211. Retrieved From: https://fearoflanding.com/accidents/title.

Yen, C-L., & Cheng, C-P. (2013). Researcher effects on mortality salience research: A meta- analytic moderator analysis. *Death Studies, 37(7),* 636–52. doi: 10.1080/07481187.2012.682290.

Zhu, X., Wang, K., Cao, A., Zhang, Y., & Qiu, J. (2020). Personality traits and negative affect mediate the relationship between cortical thickness of superior frontal cortex and aggressive behavior. *Neuroscience Letters, 718,* 1.

Index

Note: Page locators in italic refer to figures.

About the Authors

Lindsey A. Harvell-Bowman is an associate professor at James Madison University where she leads the Terror Management Lab investigating issues surrounding Terror Management Theory. Harvell-Bowman's decades of research can be found in numerous interdisciplinary journals in both psychology and communication. Harvell-Bowman is originally from Overland Park, Kansas, a member of the Osage Nation, and currently resides in the beautiful Shenandoah Valley with her husband, golden retriever, and chorkie. When she is not researching, she teaches POUND fitness classes at her local gym, enjoying the wonderful artichoke dip at the United Club at Dulles, and can often be found on a beach reading NTSB reports.

John Panetti graduated from James Madison University with a B.A. in Psychology and double minor in Communications Studies and Gender Studies. He currently works as a Community Development Analyst at ICF, doing website coordination for the Department of Housing and Urban Development.

Eric M. Wilson is a senior educator and outreach and outreach director at Wichita State University. He has more than ten years of professional experience in advertising, public relations, and journalism, specifically in the aviation industry. His research interests include airline industry public relations and media relations consulting. A former Southwest Airlines public relations intern and avid traveler, Wilson has also conducted media training for aviation managers and conducted aviation customer research in the area of airline travel. Wilson has known and commiserated about air travel with Dr. Lindsey A. Harvell-Bowman for fifteen years.

www.ingramcontent.com/pod-product-compliance
Ingram Content Group UK Ltd.
Pitfield, Milton Keynes, MK11 3LW, UK
UKHW020842290926
15470UKWH00004B/1503

9 781793 620699